Dimensions of the Cancer Problem

Dimensions of the Cancer Problem

Fikry M. Meleka

MD, Chief of Radiotherapy, Brooklyn Hospital, and Clinical Assistant Professor, Downstate Medical Center, New York, N.Y., USA

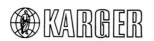 **KARGER**

1983

S. Karger · Basel · München · Paris · London · New York · Tokyo · Sydney

National Library of Medicine, Cataloging in Publication
    Meleka, Fikry M.
    Dimensions of the cancer problem
    Fikry M. Meleka. – Basel; New York: Karger, 1983
    1. Neoplasms   I. Title
    QZ 200 M519d
    ISBN 3–8055–3622–4

Drug Dosage
    The authors and publisher have exerted every effort to ensure that drug selection and dosage set forth in this text are in accord with current recommendations and practice at the time of publication. However, in view of ongoing research, changes in government regulations, and the constant flow of information relating to drug therapy and drug reactions, the reader is urged to check the package insert for each drug for any change in indications and dosage and for added warnings and precautions. This is particularly important when the recommended agent is a new and/or infrequently employed drug.

©   Copyright 1983 by S. Karger AG, P.O. Box, CH-4009 Basel (Switzerland)
    Printed in Switzerland by Effingerhof AG, Brugg
    ISBN 3–8055–3622–4

Contents

Foreword VIII

Preface IX

1   Cancer Should Concern All Segments of Society 1
     Cancer: A Concern of Society as a Whole 2

2   Cancer Initiation and the Body's Defenses 5
     Initiation of Cancer 6
        Difference between Normal and Malignant Cell Behavior 8
        Is Cancer a Systemic Disease? 9
        Multiple Tumors 10
        Spread of Tumors 11
     Body Defenses 12
        Host-Immune Response to Tumors 12
     References 15

3   Predisposing Factors in Cancer 17
     Chemicals and Cancer 17
        Chemicals in the Environment and Their Relationship to Cancer 17
        Occupational Cancer 21
     Radiation and Cancer 23
     Cigarette Smoking and Cancer 27
     Sunlight, Ultraviolet Light, and Cancer 28
     Viruses, Fungi, and Cancer 28
     Genetic and Familial Factors 29
     Nutrition and Cancer 32
        Nutrition as a Supportive Measure in Cancer Management 37
        Can We Prevent or Stop Cancer by Dieting? 43
     Stress and the Mind – Behavioral Changes and the Dilemma of Predisposing
     Factors 44
        Stress and the Mind 44
        Behavioral Changes in Cancer Patients 45
        The Dilemma of Cancer: Predisposing Factors 50
     References 50

Contents

4 Race and Socioeconomic Variations in Cancer 54
  Incidence of Cancer According to Geographic Location and Social Class 54
    Geographic Variation 54
    Social Class and Cancer 55
    Change of Cancer Incidence 56
  References 57

5 Sexuality and Self-Esteem in Cancer 58
  References 62

6 Objectives of the Drive to Control Cancer 63
  Prevention 64
  Conflict between Health and Economy 65
  Cancer Prophylaxis 66
  Increased Curability 69
  Lay Education 69
  The News Media 70
  Professional Education 72
  Propagation of Accurate Knowledge – Centers of Information 72
  Crusade against Quacks 74
  The Role of Different Organizations 76
  References 77

7 Detection of Asymptomatic Cases: Screening for Cancer 78
  Conditions Necessary for the Success of Screening Programs 79
  Cost-Effectiveness 79
  Screening for Cancer of the Breast 81
    Breast Self-Examination 81
    Physical Examination 82
    Screening by Mammography 82
    Thermography 86
  Screening for Cancer of the Cervix 86
  History of Genital Herpes Infection 88
  Screening for Cancer of the Colon 90
    Cytologic Examination 93
    Sigmoidoscopy 94
    Fiberoptic Colonoscopy 95
    Barium Enema 96
  Screening for Gastric Cancer 96
  Screening for Cancer of the Lung 97
    Sputum Cytology 98
  References 99

8   Changing Concepts in Cancer Management 101
    Assistance Provided during the Course of Management 104
        How Much Should the Patient Know about His/Her Disease? 104
    Changing Concepts about Cure and Failure 105
    The Five Goals of Radical Management 106
    Varied Rolle of Different Management Modalities 106
        Surgery 106
        Radiation Therapy 107
        Chemotherapy 109
        Immunotherapy 109
        Spontaneous Regression of Tumors 110
    References 112

9   Medical Costs of Cancer Management 113
    Health Insurance 118
    References 120

10 Returning the Cancer Patient to Society 121
    Rehabilitation 121
        The Amputee 124
        Laryngectomy 125
        Colostomy and Ileostomy 125
        Breast Cancer 127
        Problems after Penectomy 129
        Maxillofacial Radical Surgery 129
    Readjustment to Society and Work 130
        Job Discrimination 130
    Future of Long-Surviving Cancer Patients 131
    References 131

11 Pain and Suffering: The Hospice Concept 133
    Difference between Pain and Suffering 135
    The Hospice Concept 136
    References 139

    Subject Index 140

Foreword

'Dimensions of the Cancer Problem' is a long overdue and needed monograph not only for the health care professional, but also for the public at large. It bridges the gap between lay and scientific writing on the subject matter in a clear, concise, intelligible and intelligent manner. The reader will come away much better informed and open minded about 'cancer': not about its cause, or its prevention or its cure, but rather about its overall status and ramification as a disease process.

My congratulations to *Fikry M. Meleka,* a nationally known radiotherapist with a vast clinical experience, for this contribution to the literature.

Brooklyn, N.Y.

Vincent Tricomi
MD, Professor and Chairman
Department of Obstetrics and Gynecology
The Brooklyn Hospital

Preface

H. G. Wells once said the disease of cancer will be banished from life by calm, unhurrying, persistent men and women working in hospital and laboratories and the motive that will conquer cancer will not be pity nor horror, it will be curiosity to know how and why.

The cancer problem seems to be an intricate web which sometimes can be unravelled in separate threads, with care and effort, in other times, it is difficult to do so. Unfortunately, this disease is surrounded by an aura of misunderstanding and misconcepts that makes it different from other diseases. The different aspects of the problem were discussed, but no available solutions were always offered. Familiarizing ourselves with the different aspects of the problem may be one step forward. In order to eliminate the fear and for better understanding to be achieved, facts have to be realized regarding the cancer patient and various problems associated with cancer.

The book is written for professional, paraprofessional, and lay people concerned with the problem.

... to my wife Amira

Chapter 1

Cancer Should Concern All Segments of Society

The literature is replete with information about cancer, different authors addressing various of the numerous problems associated with this disease. However, each has been concerned with only one or a few of the issues involved. Consequently, to many individuals the information available is either fragmented or incomplete, probably contributing to the public's intense fear of cancer. Undoubtedly, this fear is fostered by growing publicity about the disease and its rising incidence.

That the dimensions of the problem seem to be spreading beyond their true limits is apparent, particularly to persons not closely involved or familiar with cancer's various aspects. Endeavors to change the deeply rooted fatalistic attitude most people have towards the disease are worthwhile. Cancer phobia, probably aided and abetted by detailed news reports of different predisposing factors, which alarm and confuse the lay public, is sometimes crippling and poses obstacles to the early diagnosis and treatment of cancer. In this atmosphere cancer 'quackery' flourishes, with valuable time, money, and lives lost unnecessarily.

Unfortunately, because of the complex issues involved, it is virtually impossible to single out any one causative factor in a given situation. Many associated problems impede progress to the ideal state from which all predisposing factors have been eliminated.

Clusters of cancers and populations at high risk have been and still are being identified. Methods for the early detection of cancer and the problems inherent in their general use are discussed, as are cancer prevention and prophylaxis – along with the limitations of each – as alternatives to increase the survivors of the disease. The new approach and philosophy in cancer management with multidisciplinary modalities are stressed. Also covered are its impact on the body, mind, sexuality, and emotional well-being of the patient as well as the complicated socioeconomic factors involved. Only the problems associated with management – both during and after – are explained in detail; specific cancer management is not. Healing the whole person until that person can return to his or her former place in society is emphasized along with cancer's changing image, its various behaviors, and its geographic distribution. An important aspect is the ameliorating role played by public and professional education because teaching people about cancer encourages them to seek medical help while their disease is still at a curable stage. Also, the informed patient is much easier to manage through the protracted therapy that is so characteristic of cancer management.

Cancer: A Concern of Society as a Whole

Cancer is a disease that became most prevalent during the 20th century. It was known to the ancient Egyptians; the *Ebers's Paypyrus* records swellings. And, the literature discloses sporadic cases such as the gastric carcinomas of the Napolean family.

What characterizes the space-age we live in is the dramatic rise in the incidence of cancer, a rise that approached epidemic levels during the last five decades particularly, since 1 in every 4 persons may be confronted with some form of the disease at some point in life. Perhaps the 'graying' of the population of the United States and the prolonged longevity of its people contribute to the problem. In 1920, the life expectancy of white males in the United States was 54 years. By the year 2000, about 15% of the population is expected to be at least 65 years old, which may further contribute to the problem. Other contributory factors may be the multitude of changes associated with industrialization and the sophistication of modern-day society, with its competitive high-speed life-style. In addition, ecologic changes have been fast and deep, accumulating rapidly over a relatively short period of time, making the accompanying problems so monstrous they seem unsolvable. As projected by the American College of Surgeons, cancer deaths in the 1980s will exceed those of the 1970s. As a matter of fact, cancer deaths have almost doubled over the last 35 years.

The grim picture already established needs careful and attentive handling if we are to change it. Although a breakthrough in the control or elimination of cancer does not seem imminent, a solution to the problem may not be far off. A more optimistic attitude is greatly needed and is justified by the enormous scientific efforts being expended on cancer research. The knowledge gained in cancer cellular biology and the understanding of different cancer behaviors over the last three decades is unparalleled. The monies spent and the number of specialties deeply involved in the battle against cancer on its different fronts are enormous.

Early in the 20th century there were no survivors among cancer patients; the medical profession seemed helpless against the different forms of this disease. But, the picture is changing. For example, in the 1930s, less than 1 of every 5 cancer patients lived at least 5 years. In the 1950s, 1 of every 4 cancer patients lived for 5 years or more, and in the 1970s, the 5-year survival rate was increased to 1 in every 3 cancer patients. This gain from 1 in 4 to 1 in 3 over a 30-year period represents about 50,000 persons surviving each year. Through early diagnosis and prompt treatment, an additional one-sixth of all cancer patients can be expected to survive.

In 1944 only 1.8% of cancer cases were discovered at an early stage. The frequency of early detection then rose to 27.4% of all cancers diagnosed between 1944 and 1968. Due to the lay public's greater awareness of the disease and improved diagnostic procedures, the numbers of cases detected during the early stages of cancer are expected to increase further.

As reported by the Department of Health and Human Resources, the percentage of cancer patients living at least 5 years definitely increased for 17 of 35 anatomic sites in 1970. The most dramatic improvement in survival occurred in Hodgkin's disease – from 34 to 66%. In the two most frequent cancers after cancer ot the skin – the lung and prostate – the improvement in survival was not as dramatic, rising from 7 to only 9% for cancer of the lung and from 50 to 63% for cancer of the prostate. Survival rates have also increased for cancer of the breast – from 63 to 68% – and for cancer of the colon – from 44 to 50%.

Obviously, much remains to be done. However, we must not despair. The cancer problem is very similar to past epidemics of plague, smallpox, and cholera, that wiped out entire cities at a time when the human race was defenseless against these horrors. The same fears as those of cancer today must have been present. Then the discovery of the microscope revealed the microorganisms responsible for disease. However, long before specific treatment became available, prevention helped to wipe out these microbial diseases.

Cancer is a reality all of us must learn to live with and confront. To prevent prevailing fears from becoming a nightmare difficult to control, an intelligent attitude is required. What distinguishes cancer from all other serious illnesses is the flood of associated problems, each of breathtaking complexity, whose impact goes far beyond that with which the patient and family can cope, particularly during a lengthy confrontation with the disease. As the patient looks for help, assurance, and security, he can readily find it in the immediate family. A healthy family relationship is needed to absorb the disturbing feelings that arise and is a first-line defense, sheltering the patient and shielding contacts from the turbulence of the shocking experience of cancer. The safety and integrity of the family, therefore, are essential; if the shower of new problems overwhelms that shelter, the consequences are reflected in the whole of society.

The problem seems to be mushrooming beyond its true limits, as there are many unanswered questions, due probably to the ramifications of issues and the multitude of approaches to the disease, making everyone feel it is an unsolvable enigma. Under these conditions, misunderstandings and issues must be put in proper perspective before the true dimensions of the problem are to be recognized. On the personal level, a more positive attitude as well as active participation are needed, if we are to change those deeply seated pessimistic concepts about cancer. Above all, the concerted efforts of different institutions and organizations are required. Long- and short-term planning is essential as all aspects of the problems cannot be solved overnight. Giving priority to more plausible solutions that can yield immediate benefits helps to elevate morale and change the fatalistic attitude the general public has towards cancer.

Chapter 2

Cancer Initiation and the Body's Defenses

The word cancer is derived from the latin *cancri,* meaning Crab, which connotes a very ominous disease characterized as insidiously aggressive, gradually incarcerating, and 'taking its victim by surprise'. Even the term malignant gives the impression that the body is being invaded by an uncontrolled, sneaking, and growing number of cells that behave unpredictably. Unfortunately, nothing can be done to change current terminology. The word cancer is still used as a generic term to describe a multitude of different diseases with common traits. To many, cancer is a vicious disease, and its diagnosis is considered a death sentence. An obvious weakness in current knowledge is the concept of cancer as a single disease. Unfortunately, it is a spectrum of diseases, each differing in its aggressiveness according to many variables. Also, some cancers are more malignant than others and they vary from acute in onset with rapid deterioration and widespread dissemination to a more prolonged, chronic course with slow growth and further dissemination either later or not at all. Moreover, the behavior of some cancers is more predictable than that of others.

Predisposing factors rather than etiology are known. Some of these factors are more closely linked to the disease and better known than others. Conversely, etiology may be intrinsic or extrinsic to the host. The interplay of several factors in addition to the individual's inherent suppressed immunity are believed to make the person succumb to the disease. Although cancer is not contagious, it sometimes occurs in clusters, probably because several people are exposed to the same social, environmental, or occupational predisposing factor.

The suspected factors – carcinogenic or immunosuppressive – can be summarized as follows:

(1) Chemical: These may be present as (a) pollutants in the air, water, or food, and their sources may be industrial or occupational, car fumes, pesticides, fungicides, cosmetics, or synthetics; (b) drugs, or (c) food additives and detergents.

(2) Ionizing radiation: Sources may be medical, industrial, or atomic exposure from bomb testing, warfare, or civilian use as well as cosmic ray exposure, particularly at high altitudes.

(3)   Nonionizing radiation such as ultraviolet rays.

(4)   Food constituents.

(5)   Viruses.

(6)   Fungi.

(7)   Heredity and genetics.

(8)   Hormones, both exogenous and endogenous.

(9)   Cigarettes.

(10) Precancerous conditions.

It is believed that chronic bacterial infection and chronic irritation are closely associated with carcinogenesis. Some cancers have a more defined etiology than do others, while the incidence of certain other cancers varies with culture. It is difficult to pinpoint any one agent to blame or subsequently eliminate, and there is no way to find one or all suspected carcinogens in time to safely contain them. Although genetic build-up may play a role, there is no available method to predict when cancer will occur and what preventive measure can be taken.

Initiation of Cancer

Most malignant cells arise de novo from normal cells. However, benign tumors can be transformed to malignant tumors. In the past, the frequency of this transformation was exaggerated. Similarly, malignant tumors can regress to benign ones, as occurs when a neuroblastoma regresses to a ganglioneuroma.

There is also total agreement that cancer occurs with repeated insults by one or more carcinogens, triggering changes within the cell which initiate the malignant transformation. Genetic predisposition and chemical changes within the cell or its membrane, and probable disruption of microenvironmental conditions or growth control mechanisms may play major roles in the initiating mechanism. Whether these changes occur independently or as a chain of reactions, varying in magnitude from one cancer to another, remains to be proved. If these chain reactions are prevented from proceeding before cancer starts, or if the process can be interrupted, cancer might be prevented.

Cancerous transformation of the cell involves morphologic cellular and biochemical intracellular changes. For example, the gradual morphologic changes of uterine cervical cancers begins with a progressive increase in cell dysplasia with obvious visible changes, followed sooner or later by visible precancerous changes. Similar changes – probably accompanied by other intracellular changes – have been seen in bronchial and esophageal carcinomas. However, it is not known at the present time whether the same gradual transformation occurs in other cancers as well. Nevertheless, progressive changes do occur with repeated exposure to carcinogenic insults. If they are detected in their early stages, as in cervical dysplasia, these changes can be treated and the situation reversed to normal.

The latent period for carcinogenic initiation varies with such factors as inherent predisposition, anatomic location, and other variables. Certain cellular enzymes can immediately recognize and repair the damage created by insults as soon as they occur. High blood enzyme levels in cancer patients could be related to these processes. Moreover, more than 50 years ago, the concentration of glycolytic enzymes, which are mostly anaerobic, was found to be much higher in precancerous than in normal tissue.

Enzymes play different roles in relation to cancer; some can destroy the malignant cell. The activity of the enzyme phospholipase, which is known to act on the cell membrane to affect its action, in a similar way to that of prostaglandin, as can chew the cell membrane, clearly demonstrating that the cell harbors within itself the seeds of its own destruction.

Microsomal function oxidase (MFO), an enzyme in the liver, lung, intestine, and other tissues, is usually activated by procarcinogens, influenced by other factors and enhanced by vitamins such as ascorbic acid, riboflavin, and so on. Sometimes, it is decreased by protein deficiency and antibiotics. The presence of these enzymes in the bloodstream could herald the presence of cancer.

Biochemical Intracellular Changes. Various theories have been proposed to explain the different intracellular changes associated with carcinogenesis. These changes are summarized as follows:

(1) Chemicals that interfere with cell differentiation accumulate within the cell as a result of carcinogenic insult, preventing it from developing into specialized tissue with a specific function. All cancer cells lose this characteristic of differentiation because they have no function to perform.

(2) Abnormal film formation may occur on the membrane of cells causing them to adhere to each other in an irreversible manner. The cat-

echolamines can convert a coagulated cellular system to a flocculated one and potentially trigger cancer. In general, major structural changes occur in the cell membrane of the malignant cell.

(3) Genetic mutation also can be seen as a gel-like material that forms between the two strands of DNA.

(4) Disruption of the growth control mechanism has been described by Dr. *Theodore Puck,* Professor of Biology, Physics, and Genetics at the University of Colorado. He explained that cell growth is regulated by an intracellular network of microtubules linking the cell membrane to the nucleus. If this growth control mechanism is disrupted, malignancy develops. Dr. *Brugarlos* and Dr. *Gonzales* of Spain, in their attempts to restore this disrupted growth regulatory mechanism to normal, found that thioproline reversed the malignant process of some cancers, particularly epidermoid cancer of the head and neck.

(5) Disruption of microenvironmental conditions has been described by others. A temporary shift in the local acid-base equilibrium toward alkaline may precede the formation of some gastrointestinal tumors. In fact, *Herguindy* [10], at Roswell Park Memorial Institute, reported, on the basis of animal research, that some malignant tumors can be prevented or controlled by systemic acidification. He suggested that total body acidification in animals antagonizes tumor growth, an effect that appears to be independent of starvation, ketosis, or both.

Difference between Normal and Malignant Cell Behavior

Normal cells are known to differ from malignant ones in their rate of adhesiveness and stickiness. Cancer cells are weakly adhesive as they lack the calcium usually required to maintain cellular adhesiveness. These cells seem to produce an abnormal quantity of mucopolysaccharides, which combine with calcium ions to disrupt the linkage between cells [1].

The normal cell, after mutation, acquires new characteristics. Disruptions in its cellular mechanisms and dividing capacity lead to permanent cellular defects, often with a change in doubling time from normal to one characteristic of a specific type of tumor. Further, the pattern of the cancerous tissue differs from that of the original normal tissue to a variable degree. The greater the degree of similarity between the tumor and the original pattern, the better differentiated it will be. The rate of local invasion and the incidence of distant metastases vary with the rate of differentiation. Also, it is assumed that the behavior of a tumor varies with other factors such as tumor-bed and tumor-host relationships.

Tumors of the same microscopic type, if located in different anatomic areas, behave differently and their differentiation may vary. For example, squamous carcinoma of the cervix behaves differently from squamous cell carcinoma of the lung and squamous cell carcinoma of the oral cavity which becomes less differentiated as it develops further posteriorly. For example, carcinoma of the anterior tongue is usually more differentiated than is carcinoma of the posterior third.

As stated earlier, cancer grows insidiously, forming masses of cells. Its growth, unless controlled, is endless. The tumor will grow at an appalling rate, but the doubling time of its cell cycle does not change. The tumor may reach kilograms in weight with continuous division, and its growth rate is proportional to its size. Thirty doubling times are required for a tumor to enlarge to 1 cm in diameter, at which time it contains about 1 billion cells. *Cooling and Loeffler* [5] report that a tumor with a doubling time of 60 days would reach a size of 1 cm in 5 years.

Most cancers are detected when they reach 1–10 g, except for superficial cancers, which can be detected earlier. Tumor cells, as they grow, crush the surrounding normal cells, so that they give way to the progressing cancer cell. As reported by *Baserga* [2], the invasiveness of tumor cells may be related to the proteolytic enzymes they secrete.

Cancer invades the lymphatics as emboli of tumor cells flowing with the current of lymph. If the lymph nodes in the direction of flow have been completely destroyed and replaced by tumor, lymph begins to flow in the opposite direction – retrograde permeation – to distal lymph nodes because the cells are clogged. Lymph node involvement can usually be predicted as it generally occurs in an orderly fashion without skipping a chain of lymph nodes. As the tumor grows, it replaces the lymph node cells almost completely, destroying their normal structure. The lymph nodes enlarge as the tumor grows. Knowledge of the distribution of draining lymph nodes in different anatomic areas and the predictability with which they become involved marks an improvement in what some describe as prophylactic cancer management.

Is Cancer a Systemic Disease?

Almost all cancers begin with a single cell, spread locally, and then disseminate to other organs. One cancer cell may undergo at least 30 doubling times to reach a size of 1 cm, most often without proven evidence of distant metastasis. When cancers smaller than 1 cm are located in the uterine cervix, breast, larynx, or other location, 90–95% of them can be cured by local treatment, strongly indicating that cancer starts as a local disease and not a systemic problem. Advanced cancer of the bladder and of the uterine cervix remains a local problem up to the time of the patient's death, rarely disseminating out of the pelvic area. Postmortem examinations usually reveal that these patients die of uremia and obstructive uropathy. Leukemia and multiple myeloma, where cancer cells are disseminated throughout the body, are considered systemic diseases by most investigators. Yet, studies by *Fialkow* [6], using genetic markers, to distinguish their origin – single cell or multicellular – indicated that these cancers originate from a single cell, as does Burkitt lymphoma.

Later in the course of the disease, the cancer cells disseminate throughout the body; systemic distribution may occur earlier in some tumours than in others, depending on many variables.

Multiple Tumors

Tumors may be multiple from the start, have the same or different pathology, and may occur in the same or in different organs. They may also occur simultaneously or in sequence. The incidence of simultaneous cancers is less than 4%. However, most cancers occur in a consecutive manner, even though the same cancer can occur on different areas of the skin at the same time because large areas of skin surface are exposed continuously to ultraviolet light.

Two paired organs – breast, ovaries, kidneys, and so forth – can be involved simultaneously or consecutively. *Spratt and Hoag* [15] reported that the probability cancer will develop in the second of the paired organs is above average.

Hereditary types of retinoblastomas, neuroblastomas, or Wilm's tumor are most often bilateral and usually occur at an earlier age. When cancerous tumors develop consecutively in the same patient, they have a predilection for certain organs, usually the larynx and lung or the oral cavity and esophagus, according to *Cook* [4].

Multiple cancers are being detected with increasing frequency because today's workups are more thorough and complete. Also, as more cancers are being controlled or cured, patients are living longer; one-third can be expected to develop another cancer, if they live long enough. Generally speaking, the graying of society is a contributory factor because people live long enough to survive more than one cancer.

Spread of Tumors

Tumors constantly shed cells. These cells are carried to distant organs through the bloodstream and lymph at rates that vary from one tumor to another. The fate of these tumor cell emboli is speculative. Most of the cells fail to develop into metastatic foci. The proportion that manage to survive in another location – in what is described as the site of arrest – is still unknown. Tumor cells have an affinity for, settle down in, and grow in traumatized parts in rats. This is also true for humans, according to a report by *Fischer* [7]. At these traumatized sites, tissues subsequently devitalize so that the tumor cells have a better chance of lodging and growing on their own as a sporadic focus independent of the primary tumor. Some investigators have speculated that a relationship simulating that between mother and daughter exists between the primary and widespread metastatic lesions of some tumors. This relationship has been demonstrated in adenocarcinoma of the kidney with widespread metastasis where resection of the primary renal cancer was followed by the disappearance of metastatic foci, a situation analogous to that in which killing the mother causes the daughters to die.

The *soil theory* explains the fate of tumor cell emboli. Suitable conditions for cells to settle down and grow are needed for the formation of metastatic foci. There are certain locations in which distant metastases never develop. For example, skeletal muscles never develop metastases, probably because of their increased vascularity or other factor. Only 39% of patients with circulating cancer cells develop distant metastases compared with 18% in those negative for circulating cancer cells. *Roberts et al.* [14] mentioned that 7% of 766 patients with cancer and blood positive for cancer cells had a 5-year survival rate comparable to that of patients with negative blood samples. Thus, the significance and fate of a circulating tumor cell remains an enigma. In a critical review of their study of 5,000 patients from 40 different investigative teams, *Goldblatt and Nadel* [9] found cancer cells in the bloodstream of approximately 20% of their curable patients and 30% of the incurable ones. Although cancer cells have the ability to form metastatic foci, they can also hibernate, remaining dormant or latent for variable periods without producing clinical manifestations. This period, usually de-

scribed as the lag period, varies in duration depending on host-tumor relationships.

Body Defenses

Immune defense mechanisms protect the body against the continuous
assaults and intrusions of bacteria, viruses, and tumor cells. These foreign
bodies are treated as unwelcome enemies. Hence, different defense mechanisms are launched to destroy them. The complexity of the immune mechanism parallels its highly sophisticated apparatus, which is responsible for
fighting a multitude of foreign intruders, and in this respect is truly remarkable.

The body's defense against any foreign intrusion is tremendous and
more potent at the early stages of invasion than later on. As cells begin to
multiply rapidly, the body's defenses begin to wane and outside intervention
becomes necessary to achieve the best outcome.

Historically, modern immunology began in 1959, when immune
mechanisms were found to have a potential impact on both the diagnosis
and treatment of cancer. The body can recognize malignant cellular transformation instantly, at which time the cancer cell is treated as a foreign
body. There are two or more immune responses to neoplasia, according to
Anderson and Green [1].

Host-Immune Response to Tumors

Unfortunately, a tumor burden may have to reach a critical level of invasiveness before it can provoke a detectable host reaction.

Tumor-versus-Host Response

This response is related to the characteristics and behavior of each
malignancy, which varies in its capacity to evade, deceive, and overwhelm
the body's defense mechanism. In addition, the neoplastic cell is believed to
elicit antibodies to inhibit the specific tissue antigenicity of the tumor cell
surface. Thus the tumor cell becomes anonymous to the involved tissue, and
normal tissue becomes unable to express its full antigenic potential.

The immune system is a dynamic defense mechanism in which lymphocytes of various shapes and sizes parade continuously through tissues. Each

of these lymphocytes carries a specific surface marker that varies according to the anatomic location in which it matured. Lymphocyte transformation normally occurs with the development of malignancy. However, in intraepithelial cancer of the vulva, lymphocyte transformation is less than normal, according to *Geski and Reinhelter* [8]. In addition, *Rivera* [13] reported that leukocyte migration was greatly inhibited by cervical-cancer antigen. It is obvious that shortcomings of the immune defense mechanism usually accompany the development of cancer.

The bursa of Fabricius of birds is capable of directing maturing cells to populate the lymphoid follicles, the red pulp and the germinal centers of the spleen in order to participate in the antibody and immunoglobulin system, other components of the immune mechanism. The precise location of the bursal equivalent in man has not been identified, but the site may lie in the liver, spleen, bone marrow, or gastrointestinal lymphoids. The B cells are the bursa equivalent lymphocytes that acquire morphologic and functional characteristics when they migrate to the bursa of Fabricius of avian species. Another major pathway of lymphocyte differentiation involves the maturation of stem cells into thymus-derived or T cells. These thymus-dependent cells are involved in cellular immunity and are responsible for the delayed hypersensitivity response to antigens. They are found in the paracortical areas of lymph nodes and the perivascular region of the spleen and circulate four to six times a day, accounting for 60–70% of the normal peripheral blood lymphocytes. Lymphatic cell permeation in and around the tumor indicates that a good immune response to the tumor is present. The B cells produce antibodies and are related to serum Ig levels. They are found in the follicular centers of lymphoid tissues and in the Malpighian bodies of the spleen, lamina propria of the gastrointestinal tract, and in bone marrow. B cells comprise 20–25% of the circulating peripheral lymphocytes.

The tumor behaves as an antigen, foreign to the body, and induces a reaction that results in the subsequent release of antibodies into the serum of cancer patients, similar to the delayed hypersensitivity reaction activated by lymphoid cells. The antigen-antibody complex generates an immunologic memory. The excess of tumor antigen associated with a larger tumor burden could attenuate this specific host-immune response against the tumor cell. As reported by *Kato* [12], circulating levels of the antigen of human cervical squamous cell carcinoma were found to be correlated with prognosis. There is a corresponding increase in serum antigen levels with extension of the disease. Consequently, levels drop with therapy. Hence, a defect in the immune response to tumor antigen usually precedes clinical recognition of the tumor.

Immune Hyporesponsiveness

Immune hyporesponsiveness to antigen may be related to the tumor and its ability to compromise the defense mechanism, possibly due to an inherent aggressiveness of the tumor despite the immunocompetence of the host. At other times, however, the immuno-incompetence caused by genetic disorders of the immunoregulatory mechanism has to be considered the major factor in carcinogenesis. This is why it was suggested that identifying the problem and discovering immunodeficiency early may be a step toward the early detection or prevention of cancer. Promoters and predisposing factors may help to compromise the normal immune mechanism. Age, infection, trauma, burns, stress, malnutrition, and drugs may be closely related to what is described as the fertile soil that does not prevent tumor cells from settling, dividing, and growing. We live only so long as the immune system is healthy enough to overcome the different cancers that try to develop in our bodies. *Burnett* [3] suggested that malignant cells are a common occurrence but are usually destroyed by the host's immunologic surveillance mechanism.

Tumor cells are assumed to have unique surface antigens, usually recognized by the body and immediately considered foreign to its cells. The body can then develop appropriate and effective immune responses to these antigens. As a matter of fact, cancer is considered part of the body, but lies dormant within it until host immunity is at its lowest level. Only then does the cancer begin to grow. Identifying tumor antigens early in the course of the disease may help to increase its curability. Unfortunately, unique tumor antigens have been difficult to distinguish among different human neoplasms. Therefore, progress in the field of immunotherapy has been disappointing, as is the early discovery of malignancy by the detection of specific tumor markers. Much needs to be learned about the quantitative and qualitative differences in tumor antigenicity and the identification of a spectrum in a single tumor-cell population. Marker molecules must be identified earlier in the course of a malignancy, long before the number of cancer cells reaches millions and the bulk of the disease overwhelms body defenses. The future seems promising for the identification of new markers. Consequently, radioimmunoassays of α-fetoprotein (AFP) and the β-chain of human chorionic gonadotrophin (HCG) is essential for the diagnosis, staging, and further follow-up of some testicular tumors. The monoclonal antibodies may help one to recognize and identify different tumor antigens and other marker molecules and may prove to be valuable antitumor agents. The monoclonal antibodies (hybridoma) used to detect different cancer antigens can also be used to classify different forms of cancer, detect early cancer, and reveal sites of spread.

Immunodeficiencies

Lymphatic and epithelial cancers develop with high frequency in persons with primarily genetically determined immunodeficiencies; the risk of breast cancer in these individuals is 100 times greater than that of the normal population. A large number of patients with primary immunodeficiency may develop gastrointestinal malignancies, particularly cancer of the stomach.

In addition, the incidence of cancer is high among patients who receive immunosuppressive medication – that is, recipients of renal transplants – or immunosuppressive regimens. The mortality rate is 100 times greater in these groups than in the general population. In a study at the National Cancer Institute (NCI), the risk a lymphoma will develop in recipients of renal transplants was about 35 times higher than in normal individuals. *Hoover and Fraumeini* [11] found that these tumors developed an average of 32 months after transplantation. It is possible that some of the tumors were already present at the time of transplantation. However, they became manifest in a shorter period of time.

More than one theory has been advanced to explain the unusually high incidence of lymphoma associated with immunodeficiency. Immunosuppressive drugs are believed to have a direct effect on the thymus gland, which depresses the proliferation of lymphoid tissue. Therefore, when thymic function is depressed, it has no control over lymphatic tissue. A very high incidence of cancer is found in animals with congenital immunodeficiencies and a congenitally absent thymus. Yet, data are insufficient at present to support the general concept that a faulty immunologic mechanism is common to all cases of cancer.

References

1   Anderson, M.R.; Green, H.N.: Tumor host relationship. Br. J. Cancer, N.Y. *21:* 27–32 (1967).
2   Baserga, R.: A study on the establishment and growth of tumor metastasis with tritiated thymidine. Cancer Res. *20:* 910–917 (1960).
3   Burnett, Sir McFarlane: Immunologic surveillance (Pergamon, Oxford 1970).
4   Cook, G.B.: A comparison of single and multiple primary cancers. Cancer, N.Y. *19:* 959–966 (1966).

5   Cooling, V.P.; Loeffler, R.K.: Observations on growth rates of human tumors. Am. J. Roentg., Rad. Ther. nucl. Med. *19:* 76–988–1000 (1956).

6   Fialkow, P.J.: Human tumors studied with genetic markers, birth defects in cancer and genetics book. Birth Defect Conference, vol. 12, p. 123 (Liss, New York 1975).

7   Fisher, B.: Trauma and localization of tumor cells. Cancer, N.Y. *20:* 30 (1967).

8   Geski, J.C.; Reinhelter, E.R.: Abnormalities of lymphocytes transformation in women with intraepithelial cancer of the vulva. Obstet. Gynec., N.Y. *52:* 332–336 (1978).

9   Goldblatt, S.; Nadel, E.M.: Cancer cells in the circulating blood – a critical review, Acta cytol. *9:* 6 (1965).

10   Herguindy, S.: Effects of systemic acidification of mice with sarcoma 180. Cancer Res. *39:* 4364–4371 (1979).

11   Hoover, R.; Fraumeini, J.F.: Risk of cancer in renal transplant recipient. Lancet *ii:* 55–57 (1973).

12   Kato, H.: Tumor antigen of human cervical squamous cell carcinoma – correlation of circulating level with disease progress. Cancer, N.Y. *43:* 585–590 (1979).

13   Rivera, E.: Leukocyte migration inhibition assay of tumor immunity in patients with cervical cell carcinoma. Cancer, N.Y. *43:* 2297–2305 (1979).

14   Roberts, S.S.; Hengesh, J.W.; McGrath, R.G.; Valaitis, J.; McGrew, E.A.; Cole, W.H.: Prognostic significance of cancer cells in the circulating blood – a ten year evaluation. Am. J. Surg. *113:* 757–762 (1967).

15   Spratt, J.S.; Hoag, M.G.: Incidence of multiple primary cancer. Ann. Surg. *164:* 775–784 (1966).

Chapter 3

Predisposing Factors in Cancer

Chemicals and Cancer

Chemicals in the Environment and Their Relationship to Cancer

The continuous infiltration of chemicals into the environment and its natural ecosystem was destined to be reflected in humans and in wildlife. The pollution that resulted is a man-made problem – therefore subject to his control – that poses serious threats to the continuity of life on this planet.

The environmental changes involve several aspects, among them the chemical pollution of a naturally balanced system. The present situation developed rapidly over a relatively short period of time, reaching a critical level in only a few decades. Surveys of water pollution taken in 1928 and 1929 showed no cause for concern. Later, it was thought that the developing pollution was confined to harbors and rivers near heavily industrialized areas. It was also thought that polluted waters were diluted by open currents, thereby diluting the hazards until self-purification was complete.

In 1937, fish kills attracted the attention of concerned authorities, but the people were not aware of the dangers involved and the issue did not get the concern it deserved, despite the publicity given to it. In 1949 and 1950, the gross pollution of bathing beaches was publicized.

Pollution biology began to evolve as a specialty in the 1940s. Although few pollution biologists were known at that time, their role in the evolving water bioassays were not appreciated and as a career, pollution biology was looked down upon. Workers in the field were considered sewage laborers. However, although primitive at the start, water pollution control continued to grow as a science and soon gained widespread approval. Gradually, pollution control became a national movement that lobbied to eliminate the garbage dumped by humans. That more aggressive measures were needed was evident in 1949 when steps were taken to prevent the discharge of municipal sewage in an attempt to protect the health of people and terminate a public nuisance.

Modernization continued to disfigure the environment, and it soon became clear that industrialization, which partly led to the population explosion, both were the main causes of most environmental problems. The present crisis erupted suddenly largely because of the lay public's ignorance of the causes and consequences of the changes accumulating. Later, indifference and economic greed became the leading causes.

Long-standing neglect was apparent, with repeated oil spills in water and the accumulation of such hazards as mercury, PCBs, asbestos, kepone, as well as acid drainage from coal mines and other industries. Unconventional problems like the widely publicized Legionnaire's Disease that has baffled scientists for so long have increased the public's apprehension. The ineffectiveness of human capabilities in foreseeing or handling different environmental crises was clearly evident. Environmentalists were characterized as trying to preserve nature by applying pressure and loudly denouncing those responsible for pollution, and were not totally successful in solving the problem.

In the middle and late 1960s, the rapid expansion of different movements designed to prevent pollution was unprecedented. The complexity of the issues involved was obvious. Toxic wastes as well as such metals as mercury, lead, copper, and even spilled radioactive materials became part of the problem. Not only was industry to blame but so was the domestic use of detergents and the medicinal use of fluorine and chlorine. However, a mere change in environment to divert its natural course created problems that had detrimental effects, not directly related to cancer.

Dams on rivers, for example, can create problems when the rapid spill of water from a height to the depth of the river traps air in the water, increasing the concentration of dissolved nitrogen under pressure to the point of supersaturation. The nitrogen-supersaturated water causes Bubble Disease, which results in the loss of millions of fish and therefore millions of dollars. In a study of the Snake River, about 2 million adult fish are expected to be lost during the period 1976 to 2000 [19] for an economic loss of from $ 47.2 million to $ 126.9 million unless some action is taken. This problem can be remedied by modifying the structure of the dam.

In addition, increasing amounts of organic sediments, a high water temperature, and poor water circulation deplete the concentration of dissolved oxygen available to fish. Consequently, the fish become hypoxic, their metabolism slows, and they accumulate toxins. Even the thermal changes produced by power plants are lethal to fish. Furthermore, changes in the salinity and pH value of the water can change its osmotic pressure, subjecting the fish to even greater stress. Harm was first inflicted on other nonhuman species so that very little attention was given to the problem.

Nature and marshes were supposed to take care of most of the waste. But minerals are particularly difficult to dispose of and are usually passed on to fish, then to birds and whales, and finally to humans. The contamination of fish by toxic waste may be directly or indirectly related to the problem in humans and is a good example of how different hazardous chemicals or environmental changes affect the lives of different creatures as a whole. The high levels of methyl mercury recently found in fish [40] can remain in their bodies for several years after the polluting source has been eliminated. Consequently, accumulations of mercury have been found in fish predators such as mink and other animals [14].

Lead, cadmium, and other metallic organic compounds as well as other pollutants have also been detected in high concentrations in fish. The toxicity of these pollutants and their effects on fish have been predicted by different bioassays. A working hypothesis has been formulated to forecast such incidents as humans are also subject to the same pollutants. Even the air we breathe is also affected by different spraying operations: insecticides, herbicides, defoliants, car and plane fumes, as well as several other hazards, all of which form a wide spectrum of possible carcinogens.

Most of the time, carcinogenicity affecting humans could be traced to several obvious causes, and can be assessed on different occasions by the following methods:

(1) Extrapolation of data on carcinogenicity obtained from studies in different animal species to humans. This in itself is a problem because extrapolation may lack specific answers to specific problems.

(2) Accidental exposure to pollutants such as agent orange in Vietnam, contaminants of dioxin and TCCD in timber and railroad workers, and the dumping problems of the Love Canal with their known mutagenic effects.

(3) Occupational and environmental increase in the incidence of cancer.

The question of carcinogenesis has begun to preoccupy scientists, the general public, and officials of different agencies. People have become so frightened that they are beginning to wonder if there is a safe place on earth for them to live in. Others believe we are virtually swimming in a sea of carcinogens and live with the uneasy feeling that we are playing a game of chance, each of us waiting for the time bomb to drop and makes each of us a cancer statistic in sequence.

The EPA has estimated that 50,000 chemicals are in common use, not including drugs and food additives. The public in general feels enough is not being done about the disposal of chemical carcinogens, particularly in view of the rising incidence of cancer. Unfortunately, toxic waste disposal is a profitable business, one usually handled by people who are either unaware of or unconcerned with the devastating consequences of improper disposal. Moreover, 60% of the materials dumped are chemical carcinogenic or teratogenic waste.

In the United States dumping sites are underestimated at about 50,000; only 10% are known to be safe. And, the money needed to clean up all dumping sites may amount to $ 40 billion. Complicating the problem is the issue of rising cost-effectiveness, a thorny subject to the extent that cost-effect overshadows concern for a worker's health and the welfare of all people. Although the cost of environmental regulation may amount to $ 100 billion per year, this sum represents less than 3% of the gross national product (GNP). Moreover, industry claims that the present regulations impose different standards and on the whole are confusing and difficult to comply with. Unfortunately, few chemicals have been tested for their carcinogenic potential and their safe concentrations are unknown. Also, very little is known about the effect of other chemicals. In 1976, the National Institute of Occupational Safety and Health's (NIOSH) registry of the toxic effects of chemicals contained over 22,000 substances; only 1900 of these were known to be carcinogenic by in vivo laboratory tests. No one knows for certain the latency period between the onset of exposure to a specific chemical carcinogen and the time cancer develops. Most often, it is estimated to average about 10 to 20 years, varying according to the intensity and duration of exposure and other vaguely defined biologic factors.

Solutions are either difficult to find or the problems are difficult to solve. For example, eliminating the nitrites known to be carcinogenic and used as preservatives in meat may cause many deaths from botulism. Unfortunately, there is no effective substitute for nitrites at the present time. Also, locating safe dumping sites always meets with resistance in different communities, and decision makers always try to locate a prison or mental institution or even a safe dumping site 'in someone elses backyard'.

In a 1960 and later studies, *Higginson* [26] estimated that 70–90% of all human cancers are likely to be caused by environmental factors. For the years 1970–1976, the incidence of cancer was estimated to have increased by 10%. *Fraumeni* [21] estimated that 30–40% of cancers in the United States are categorized as high risk which can be prevented. Some went even further, stating that if we could identify and subsequently eliminate different hazardous agents, we may then be able to wipe out cancer. But the changes are so deep, even genetic causes of familial cancer are thought to be influenced by environmental changes.

At present, most authorities believe that environmental causes of cancer are more crucial than genetic or racial causes. The incidence of cancer in most immigrants tends to shift from the rate in their original countries to that of residents indigenous to the host country.

Occupational Cancer

The first known expression of concern about occupational hazards was stated by a German physician who in 1472 described the 'evil of vapors of lead' and the irritating fumes of other metals such as mercury, to which goldsmiths were exposed. The first chemical reports of an occupational carcinogen was made by *Percivill Port,* who described cancer of the scrotum among chimney sweeps in England, caused by exposure to carbon soot and hydrocarbons. *Siegel* [44] reviewed the development of the uses of mercury and reported an increasing awareness of its toxicity.

A survey conducted by NIOSH from 1972 to 1974 estimated that approximately 1% of the total working population (900,000) were exposed to one or more carcinogens. The Department of Health, Education and Welfare reported that 1.5–2.5 million workers may be exposed to asbestos alone. Yet, occupational hazards are suspected to cause 1–5% of all cancers. Cancer alleys, in which the death rate from cancer is above the national average, began to appear in the United States, as shown in the National Cancer Mortality Analysis. Some suspect that this problem is far greater than it seems because the mutagenic effect of these hazards could be latent and not yet accounted for. However minimal the carcinogenic effect, different studies indicate there is a potentiating effect between different carcinogens, as the incidence of cancer among factory workers is higher in smokers than nonsmokers.

Both the Occupational Safety and Health Administration (OSHA) and NIOSH work together to define and enforce allowable concentrations of carcinogens to which workers can be exposed. A threshold level value (TLV) for only 17 chemical carcinogens has been issued, but these concentrations are arbitrarily evaluated and could be changed at any time. An attitude that permits a certain level of exposure risk is difficult to accept without reservation. Unfortunately, these matters were not openly discussed in factories because of the responsibilities involved and the fear of warning workers or the public of the potential risk from exposure to these chemicals. Even available medical care is not clearly defined and little information is offered. However, in all fairness it must be said that sometimes the evidence needed to prove or disprove the carcinogenicity of chemicals is hard to extrapolate from animal studies alone, and these studies are very time-consuming. Consequently, scientific evaluations are necessary before the matter becomes a public issue. If the problem is publicized before it is well defined, no one will accept responsibility because of the liability involved. Investigations, therefore, may be impeded and the facts hidden. Too much publicity about clusters of cancer in certain geographic locations or of chromosomal damage and birth defects could trigger fear and anxiety. This situation could be exploited by extremists and opportunists to discredit authorities and to increase lagging confidence in them. Unfortunately, the time is ripe to promote their ideas and merchandise.

The Department of Health and Human Service usually sets guidelines for the intramural use of different concentrations of chemicals, replacing them with less carcinogenic or with noncarcinogens. Adequate ventilation and dust control mechanisms can be used to decrease airborne hazards. Protective clothing and devices conforming to regulatory guidelines for waste disposal are usually available.

Chemicals are usually recognized as carcinogens only when they possess initiating and promoting activities. They have to be metabolized in the body before they ultimately become carcinogens actively involved in the induction of tumors.

The induction of human cancer is thought to be a multistage process. The first stage is initiation, which is both irreversible and mutagenic in nature, occurs rapidly, and results in one or more mutations of cellular DNA. The initiated cell is not a tumor cell.

The second stage is the promoter stage, which must be prolonged and probably involves more than one process. Affected cells, prompted by promoter agent, develop into tumor cells. This process is reversible if doses of promoter are too low or too widely spaced. The tumor does not develop unless the initiator or the promoter is administered in appropriate doses [36]. Furthermore, tumors do not develop if the promoting agent is applied before rather than after the initiating agent. Different initiators and promoters vary in their potency, while a complete carcinogen is one that possesses both initiating and promoting activity.

The third stage is progression of cancer.

Radiation and Cancer

The biologic as well as the harmful effects of X-rays became known not long after they were discovered in the late 19th century [3]. Historically, the Becquerel burn helped to reveal the effect of X-rays on human tissue. Different skin cancers and an increased incidence of leukemia were found among radiologists who used radiation without taking precautions, probably because they were not fully aware of the hazards involved. Among the survivors of the atomic bomb dropped on Hiroshima, Japan, the incidence of cancer was definitely increased. At the present time, concern about the potential carcinogenic effects of radiation is widespread. To the layman, radiation is almost synonymous with cancer. As one of the most thoroughly studied carcinogen, there are many reports of its effects in the literature.

The sources of radiation may be natural or manmade. Natural sources are cosmic rays, natural radioactive materials, and isotopes in the earth's crust. The level of radiation from natural sources to which all people are exposed is known as background radiation. Flying in airplanes at high altitudes, or mountain climbing increases an individual's exposure to cosmic rays. Ozone has a potentiating effect on cosmic radiation. Sources of manmade radiation cause most radiation hazards and can be summarized as follows:

(1) Exposure to atomic bomb radiation, including repeated atomic tests.

(2) The use of atomic energy for civil purposes and energy production in different industries.

(3) Medical use of radiation.

The civilian use of atomic energy is a controversial subject, especially since energy demands all over the world are expected to increase in the next 5 to 10 years. The demand cannot be met with oil alone and countries will have to rely on atomic energy, which has its opponents and proponents and is a very sensitive political issue. With the recent energy crisis, oil prices soared, clearly indicating that the continued dependence on energy produced from oil is very inflationary. Moreover, the technologies and facilities available to develop more nuclear energy in the United States, further complicate the problem. Energy self-sufficiency, with the absence of air pollution caused by burning coal, would be advantageous, and a plus in favor of nuclear energy. The most serious problem is nuclear waste-dumping and the unfortunate accidents that can occur, such as that at the Three-Mile Island and other nuclear plants.

Radiation exposure during medical use has been studied and reported in a 2,000-page treatise submitted to the Interagency Task Force on Health Effects of Ionizing Radiation. People adversely exposed to radiation were closely reviewed and the results studied [2]. Necessary steps to reduce the harmful effects of radiation exposure were suggested. The Task Force concluded that significant exposure from man-made radiation occurs during diagnostic and therapeutic medical examinations. This diagnostic use of X-rays and radiopharmaceuticals contributes to 18 million exposure person rems each year to the population of the United States, a figure that approaches the background radiation estimated for each person as 200 millirems per year. The Task Force found that the amount of exposure caused by radiation for medical reasons is higher than expected. Consequently, a policy council (RPC) was established by President Carter in an attempt to reduce exposure to ionizing radiation and implement the recommendation of the Interagency Task Force, which is designed to determine the most effective procedure to decrease radiation hazards. As part of the careful scrutiny of opportunities to reduce medical exposure, the practice of defensive medicine, which became popular with the rise in malpractice suits, was targeted as one of the main sources of increased exposure.

A good general policy needs to be formulated to reduce medical exposure to radiation through X-ray examinations without reducing the medical benefits derived. If every physician who uses radiation procedures would familiarize him- or herself with basic radiation biology and the risks involved, unnecessary medical exposure of patients would be curtailed markedly. Unfortunately, many physicians have X-ray equipment in their offices and use this equipment, although they are not radiologists, to improve patient care. In many cases the physician is unaware of the risks involved, or considers the hazards insignificant, chiefly because it takes at least 20 years for the carcinogenic effects of radiation exposure to appear. Qualified, licensed technicians must be made to keep abreast of new techniques and the risks involved. At present, the Environmental Protection Agency (EPA) regulates medical and dental X-ray examinations and is responsible for public safety and for supervising the exposure of professionals and paraprofessionals. The EPA also enforces laws that require faulty machines be corrected or eliminated if, after inspection, they do not comply with FDA standards.

About 30% of the 278 million diagnostic X-ray procedures performed in 1979 may not have been necessary. This number is increasing at the rate of 4% per year; this means that 7 of every 10 Americans are unnecessarily exposed to medical X-rays each year. The practice of hospital admission examinations also contributes to the high incidence of unnecessary X-ray exposure.

Certain procedures have already been discontinued and are no longer recommended such as X-ray surveys for the detection of tuberculosis, which should be limited to workers in high-risk occupations – coal miners, asbestos workers, and so forth [5]. The patient can help by not asking for or insisting on certain procedures, thereby helping to reduce the overuse of X-ray examinations.

Another aspect of the overuse of X-rays is the financial implications; the total annual cost is over $ 6 billion. Insurance companies can help to reverse the trend toward increased utilization of X-ray examination by revising their reimbursement procedures. The major point of the Libassi report was that opportunities to reduce unnecessary X-ray exposure be scrutinized. To achieve this goal, the Bureau of Radiological Health (BRH) supplies required information.

Certain routine procedures such as abdominal examinations should be regulated to safeguard women who might be pregnant against exposure. The examinations should only be carried out during the first 10 days after the onset of menses – the 10-days rule. Unfortunately, this guideline is not strictly adhered to in the United States as it is in European countries. Surveys have shown that each year 300000 pregnant woman in the United States receive abdominal X-ray examinations with direct exposure to radiation. Regretably, any exposure after the start of pregnancy, particularly during organogenesis in the first 3 months of gestation when different organs are beginning to form, may lead to anomalies and may be dangerously mutagenic [42]. The fetus that receives 0.3–0.6 rad during an abdominal examination runs a high risk of leukemia, the incidence of which is increased by 50% – rising from 10 per 10000 to 15 per 10000 live births.

The American Cancer Society, in early February 1972, elected to support 12 Breast Cancer Detection Demonstration Projects, giving them an opportunity to collaborate with the NCI to enforce a 1971 act that requested state and other health agencies cooperate in establishing programs for the early detection, prevention, and treatment of cancer. However, in 1976 *Bailar* [2] published his report demonstrating the potential increase in the incidence of cancer with the increased use of mammography, making the procedure a controversial one. The effect of this controversy on the lay public as well as on physicians was a remarkable decrease in the numbers of mammograms done in 1976 – much fewer than in 1971. This decrease, due to fear primarily, also became apparent in other radiologic examinations. Nevertheless, the overall number of X-ray studies still being done is considered excessive and needs to be reduced further.

Boice and Stone [8] studied radiation exposure with mammography and its relation to breast cancer for the Environmental Epidemiology Branch of the National Institutes of Health, Bethesda, Md. He found that radiogenic breast cancer occurs after a latent period of at least 5 years in patients exposed during adolescence. With 1 rad delivered to the breast, the risk increased to about 254 to 400 excess cancer cases per 1 million women, raising the incidence of breast cancer from 7.58 to 7.61%. The cancer death rate related to X-ray exposure lies in the range of 1000 per year. But the problem of gene mutations in future generations is not accounted for.

In a second study, it was estimated that 0.5–1.4% of cancer deaths – 750–2300 excess cancer deaths – are expected to occur in 1 million people exposed once during their lifetime to 10 rad of low-level radiation. In general, the smaller the dose, the less likely cancer will develop. Certainly, 10 rad is far greater than the amount of radiation encountered daily by the population as a whole. However, the national average exposure is 0.1 rad per year, most of which comes from natural sources of radioactivity as well as dental and medical X-ray examinations, for a total of 0.2 rad.

The 1980 *Beir* report [3] stressed that cancer induced by radiation is only detectable statistically. However, cancer affecting any given patient cannot be solely attributed to radiation as opposed to other causes of cancer. Human data for radiation carcinogenesis were obtained in large part from studies in which high doses were administered. The cancer incidence-radiation exposure curve is linear only at high dosage levels, i.e., the greater the radiation exposure, the higher the incidence of cancer. However, at a level of radiation below 50 rad, the slope of the curve is no longer linear but curves gradually. Hence the incidence of cancer no longer parallels the dose of radiation. At this point it is almost impossible to extrapolate information that could be used to assess the carcinogenic rate of a level of radiation below 50 rad.

The American College of Surgeons recommended the guidelines set forth by the American College of Radiology in which a baseline mammogram is recommended for women between the ages of 35 and 40 years; age is of primary importance in the development of later complications. For women over 50 years of age, a yearly mammogram is recommended. Also recommended is the elimination of routine annual chest X-ray examinations in smokers over 40 years of age because these examinations have no effect on either the incidence of or the mortality from cancer of the lung. Johns Hopkins, Sloan Kettering, and the Mayo Clinic Hospitals reacted strongly to these recommendations because they had not yet completed their studies. Obviously, it is difficult to reconcile differences in the views of various groups, particulary those of the epidemiologists and the treating physicians, on the various issues of cancer. Such open conflicts as these tend to confuse the public, particularly when premature, presumptuous reports are involved.

The American College also does not recommend barium enema examinations be used routinely to detect colorectal cancer. Doses of radiation from nuclear diagnostic studies are also becoming a matter of concern. The same hazards exist in certain professions as exist for hospital workers who deal with radiation and for workers in nuclear reactor plants or uranium mines because they are exposed to higher levels of radiation than that received by the population as a whole.

Cigarette Smoking and Cancer

In the United States, the number of smokers had grown to around 64 millions in 1979. After leveling off for several years, this number again has started to increase, making it evident that fear tactics failed to dissuade people – particularly female teenagers – from smoking. Apparently it was easier to caution people against starting to smoke than to persuade them not to continue to smoke.

It is difficult to determine the exact population exposed to cigarette smoke, since large numbers of people are passively exposed. In 1980 cigarette smoking killed 346000 Americans and contributed to one-fourth of all cancer deaths in women [46, 52, 60]. In fact, smokers have a 10 times greater chance of developing lung cancer than nonsmokers. Some even claim that 30–35% of all cancers may be the direct result of cigarette smoking with the risk highest in those who begin to smoke at an early age. From 20 to 40% of all deaths from cancer are related to overnutrition and 1–2% to the overconsumption of alcohol. The mortality rate from cancer is eight times greater in smokers than in nonsmokers.

Smoking is also related to an increased risk of cancer of the lungs, bladder, kidney, and the head and neck. Cigarette smoking increases the risk of lung cancer, particularly in those exposed to other occupational hazards [60]. But, gloomy statistics never deterred anyone from smoking.

Studies among coal miners comparing smokers with nonsmokers made it abundantly clear that mining with its exposure to dust cannot be solely incriminated as the cause of the increased incidence of cancer in this group. To protect them against cancer requires more than just protecting them against coal dust; persuading miners to stop smoking has proved to be more effective. Legislation forbidding miners to smoke would probably be difficult to enforce, but hiring nonsmokers only may partially solve the problem. The increased risk in these groups may also be related to other personal habits and life-styles in addition to nonoccupational environmental factors; genetic background, age, and sex may also play determinant roles [60].

How effective the new low nicotine–low tar cigarettes are in reducing the incidence of cancer is not yet known.

Sunlight, Ultraviolet Light, and Cancer

That ultraviolet radiation can cause skin cancer has been discussed in detail by *Blum* [6]. However, *Unna* [51] first noted this relationship in 1894. The skin changes leading to cancer are common in sailors, outdoor workers, and sunbathers, and normally increase with age. The problem is directly related to certain wavelengths of the ultraviolet rays. At wavelengths shorter than 3,200 Å, which are more concentrated in certain geographic locations, an increased incidence of cancer of the skin is expected. Chronic exposure is an important element in inducing carcinogenesis, and certain races are prone to skin cancer. The presence or absence of skin pigments may play a decisive factor.

Viruses, Fungi, and Cancer

For over 70 years viruses have been incriminated both directly and indirectly in the etiology of malignant tumors through their suppression of immunologic mechanisms. At the time, they are known to have carcinogenic potential as they are suspected of being responsible for coincidental cellular changes and chromosomal aberrations. However, their role in genetics will be discussed later. Viruses are also implicated in X-ray oncogenesis; some researchers theorized that X-ray exposure may directly activate a dormant oncovirus. Undoubtedly, X-ray cause direct gene mutation. Similarly, it has been speculated that the carcinogenic effect of hormones occurred through a direct oncogenic virus interaction.

Viruses can be detected in tumor cells by electron microscopy. In addition, a cell-free infiltrate from a chicken with erythroblastic leukemia when injected into a normal chicken soon activated a sequence of events that ended in a similar pathologic condition. The oncogenic RNA tumor viruses, which contain reverse transcriptase, have been shown to cause neoplasia in animal models. Also, new evidence from several laboratories all over the world is implicating the venereal herpes virus as an etiologic agent for squamous cell carcinoma of the cervix. Moreover, preliminary data from these and other investigations are being studied for the possible development of a vaccine to a herpes simplex virus type 2 (HSV-2) surface antigen.

EBV (Epstein-Barr virus) was the first oncogenic virus suspected in the etiology of Burkitt's lymphoma. An oncogenic virus was also suspected to be the cause of nasopharyngeal carcinoma, in which malignant cells were shown to contain complete viral genomes [9]. Even recent epidemiologic studies strongly suggest that primary hepatocellular carcinoma (PHC) is linked to chronic viral hepatitis (HBV), as suggested by Dr. *Baruch Blumberg* and *Thomas London* [7]. Clusters of Burkitt's lymphoma and the familial spread of Hodgkin's disease have also been linked to virus, but at times environmental conditions have been suspected. That a promoter may play a role in stimulating a dormant viral infection to develop into a malignancy is always doubtful. These promoters vary for different cancers, but in Burkitt's lymphoma malaria is suspected to prepare lymphoid cells for the oncogenic effect of EBV. The virus-induced malignancy has all of the characteristics of a spontaneous tumor.

Certain fungi were also suspected of playing a role in carcinogenesis. Some suppressed the response to phytohemagglutinins in guinea pigs. Fungi were also isolated from the home of a couple who developed acute monocytic leukemia within 5 months of each other. At the same time, none of the fungi isolated from a control house nearby caused the problem. Interestingly, an increased incidence of mycostatic-producing species of fungus has been isolated from the homes of leukemia patients. However, results are still inconclusive relative to a definitive role for fungi in carcinogenesis.

Genetic and Familial Factors

The role genetic factors play in carcinogenesis is still unclear and controversial; different theories have been proposed since 1914 [4, 30, 35, 37, 41]. Tumors were found to occur most frequently in successive generations of certain families of mice, but no single genetic factor could be isolated as the responsible one for this phenomenon. All neoplastic growths were believed but not proved to have a hereditary basis. The question of whether genetic mutation or predisposition made certain individuals more susceptible to certain environmental carcinogens was never clearly answered because nongenetic factors may influence the outcome. Experimentally, there are genetic factors – inherited or acquired during life – that can influence the acceptance or rejection of tumors, favoring the genetic theory of tumor susceptibility. Defective antibody production which may have a genetic basis, may be the cause. Also, immunodeficiency may be induced genetically or acquired through the action of drugs or some other factor.

Although on the whole, constitutional genetic anomalies are associated with a low cancer risk, there is a noticeable association between certain tumors and specific chromosomal aberrations. Some hereditary diseases carry an increased risk for childhood cancers. Deletion of the 13D chromosome is always found in bilateral hereditary retinoblastoma and, as shown by HLA markers, cancer susceptibility is linked to a short arm of chromosome 6, a finding reported by Dr. *R.A. Gatti* of the University of California in Los Angeles to the American Association for Cancer Research. Common HLA haplotypes have been found in families with a high incidence of breast cancer, chronic lymphocytic leukemia, and ovarian carcinoma.

A growing body of evidence links certain genes to cancer susceptibility, and the goal of identifying cancer-susceptible genes in man is slowly being realized [25, 61]. Specialists advise cytogenetic studies in all children with congenital anomalies so as to identify gene carriers. These studies are especially important in the prenatal period as there is a 50% probability that the tumor will be transmitted to the offspring. In Down's syndrome, the incidence of leukemia is 18 times greater than in the normal population, compared to survivors of Hiroshima in whom the incidence is 1 in 60 and to persons with ankylosing spondylitis where the incidence is 1 in 270 [61].

The role of viruses relative to chromosomal defects makes it even more difficult to speculate as to whether chromosomal defects are acquired or inherited. The oncogenic theory proposes that oncogenic viruses are an integral part of the genetic material received from parents, or they may be acquired by the conventional mechanism in which a virus infects an intact cell. Theoretically, viruses remain dormant within the cell and only reveal their oncogenic nature after they became activated. Because of better management, large numbers of cancer survivors are transmitting their mutated genes to their offspring. In some of the familial diseases, environmental effects should also be considered. Individuals at increased risk for chemical carcinogenesis are thought to have a basic genetic predisposition for cancer [41, 61].

Genetic disorders may impair the host's ability to destroy spontaneously generated malignant cells. However, chemicals and viruses have additive immunosuppressive effects; both work together to compromise immunity. In immunodeficient persons, the risk of malignancy is 10,000 times higher than the 2% to 10% risk in a control population. Of these cancers, 60% will develop in the lymphoreticular system. Associated with almost each type of immunodeficiency is a characteristic malignancy.

'Cancer families' have hereditary as well as nonhereditary trends, but in all cases the incidence of adenocarcinoma of the colon, uterus, breast, and gastrointestinal tract is increased [25, 32, 50]. Age at onset is usually a decade or two earlier than observed with comparable neoplasms. Multiple primaries, most often of the colon and uterus, developed in 14% of the members of these families. Perhaps surveillance and early detection may be effective in these families and the approximate risk calculated. Therefore, it is important to identify the different cancer families and carry out predigree studies. These families are increasing in numbers because persons who have had Wilm's tumor or other pediatric malignancy are living longer. Inherited mutation depends on the penetrants for these traits. In Wilm's tumor, the rate of penetrants is only 63%, meaning that 37% of family members may carry the gene without developing the tumor. In families at high risk for cancer of the breast, a 20% incidence rate was observed – three times that in other families. An autosomal dominant gene on chromosome 10 is suspected. Some believe that 15–30% of breast cancers are genetically caused, with higher risks in close relatives, varying with age at onset, and characterized by bilateral disease. The incidence of bilateral disease varies almost twofold in postmenopausal women. However, if bilateral disease occurs in premenopausal women, risks to their relatives becomes much higher, probably tenfold higher.

Henry T. Lynch [32], in his review of familial factors in cancer of the bladder, reported that although a family relationship to bladder cancer is suspected, yet many members of such families are more exposed to other various carcinogens at the same time. He recommended that all members of families in these high-risk categories, who are particularly exposed to carcinogens, be followed carefully with routine urinalyses and cytologic examinations. The same precautions apply to families with familial disease of the colon.

In leukemic family aggregates, several generations of siblings will be affected; the incidence of leukemia among them is usually higher than that in the general population. Neonatal leukemia has also been observed and half the patients had chromosomal defects that tended to disappear during remissions and reappear during relapses. A viral factor may be involved in neonatal leukoneogenesis. Twins, particularly those of the same sex and monozygous, are known to develop leukemia either simultaneously or within 1 year of each other, suggesting an additional environmental factor is operative, according to *Gunz and Veale* [25]. As a matter of fact, the etiology of leukemia seems to be multifactorial, with interactions between hereditary and genetic predisposition added to environmental factors [61]. Both hereditary and nonhereditary factors may be involved in other tumors such as Wilm's. However, familial aggregates with an increased incidence of intestinal carcinoma but without a well-defined genetic syndrome are also known. The incidence was higher in members with blood group A and lower in those with blood group O. In some instances, a genetic defect in T lymphocytes was also suspected, as in the famous Napoleon family where grandfather, father, Napoleon himself, and each of his three sisters developed cancer of the stomach.

The cancer family syndromes are known to have a familial adenomatous polyposis with an autosomal dominant mode of inheritance; 80% of family members develop cancer. Esophageal cancer occurs in an hereditary manner in families with tylosis, a high incidence of achalasia, and Plummer-Vinson disease, which, in females, is associated with vitamin deficiency. Genetic counseling is required for siblings of involved parents and in unaffected family members to detect gene carriers.

Cytogenetic studies may reveal etiologic factors in malignant transformation [30]. And, as knowledge of the human gene map increases, changes in affected chromosomes may be related to biochemical abnormalities in the malignant cell [35]. These studies should shed light on the manner in which selected cells proliferate through malignant transformation, aid in the precise classification of these diseases, and help in designing more specific forms of therapy [37, 41].

Nutrition and Cancer

Food and its role in carcinogenesis have recently been receiving a great deal of publicity. As a natural requirement for maintaining life, food provides the ingredients essential for building the body physically and maintaining different bodily functions. Foods provide more than 50 of the nutrients needed by different systems to perform various activities [28, 54, 58]. Naturally, the body's immunologic defenses are among the recipients of these nutrients, the essential constituents of which are proteins, fats, carbohydrates, vitamins, and minerals. Unfortunately, other chemicals and contaminants are ingested with food. These contaminants are either naturally present or develop during food processing or – like fungi – during food storage. Some constituents are considered nutritive but even an excess of these may not be carcinogenic in themselves but help to create conditions that promote carcinogenesis. The main function of other constituents, such as fiber, may be essentially protective and not necessarily nutritive. Food additive, such as nitrosamines, are known to be carcinogenic. As epidemiologists have speculated, not only are contaminants harmful but essential food ingredients also have their impact. The role of some nutritional ingredients in vegetables, fruits or corn oil and some ingested chemicals was found to play a dual role in cancer. Not only do they induce the activity of certain enzymes (microsomal function oxidase) but they are capable of activating some procarcinogens. The balance between these two antagonistic reactions determines the direction of the two opposing trends. What influences the intensity of either reaction is unknown.

Overeating has been associated with an increased incidence of cancer. Similarly, undernourishment may also have a bearing on cancer incidence [21, 48]. Cooking and eating habits vary according to race. For example, the incidence of nasopharyngeal carcinoma in the Far East is high because of an excessive intake of hot and spicy food. Cancer of the stomach, pancreas, liver, and colon are also closely associated with the kinds of food ingested. Even other cancers not related to the gastrointestinal tract are also influenced by food, such as breast cancer which is known to be associated with the Western diet [53, 54, 58, 59].

The relationship of diet to the development of cancer has been studied in different animals. A deficiency or imbalance of essential nutrients has a profound effect on the induction, growth, metastasis and spread of malignant tumors. A restricted caloric intake by underfeeding genetically susceptible mice reduced the incidence of cancer, delayed the appearance of spontaneous tumors and subsequently prolonged the life span of the mice [48]: Caloric restriction in these mice also influenced the appearance of carcinogenic-induced tumors. Caloric deficiency in animals has also been consistently associated with a marked reduction in the incidence and delay in the appearance of spontaneous mammary adenocarcinoma, spontaneous hepatoma, primary lung adenocarcinoma, and spontaneous leukemia. The same results have been noted in carcinogen-induced skin neoplasia, ultraviolet-induced skin tumors, and carcinogen-induced sarcomas [27]. The decreased incidence, growth, and metastatic spread of tumors could be achieved in animals with pure protein deficiency or a deficiency of certain essential amino acids. Anecdotal reports in humans with malignant melanoma, who were treated with a phenylalanine-tyrosine restricted diet, described primary tumor growth regression, cessation of metastatic spread, and improvement in other subjective parameters.

Copeland and Dudrick [12] who studied starvation in cancer patients, postulated that malnutrition could be of potential benefit. They assumed that serum-blocking antibodies become increasingly depressed out of proportion to the depression of cell-mediated immunity, leading to a situation in which the body is better able to fight off invading cells. Others believe that starvation retards the growth of tumor cells, since overnutrition accelerates their growth rate. Although the growth of transplanted tumors was temporarily impeded in nutritionally depleted animals, the net weight of tumors in protein-depleted and well-nourished animals was essentially the same. Tumor weight to body weight ratio did not differ between nutritionally replenished animals and those that continued to receive a protein-depleted diet [12].

The claim that starvation may improve a patient's condition would be valid only if the tumor is isolated from the rest of the body. Tumor bulk and circulating cells make cancer a part of the entire body. A more plausible hypothesis is that what affects the tumor influences the entire system and compromises other functions as well. The nutritional needs of normal cells are greatly affected at a time when the added burden of the tumor's presence seriously interferes with available nutrients for normal cells; thus nutritional deprivation is aggravated further. Furthermore, the therapeutic ratio for the difference between normal and malignant cell tolerance is narrowed. During management of cancer patients, malnutrition was found to be harmful, as cachectic patients had a narrower safe therapeutic margin and results were compromised. Conversely, as the patient's nutritional status improves, the number of resting tumor cells in the G_o phase of the cell cycle, which is the most resistant phase for cell killing, will ultimately decrease. The well-nourished cells will proceed through different phases of the cell cycle, which are more susceptible to cell killing. Most important, good nutrition improves the patient's sense of well-being, increases his resistance to infection, and accelerates his recovery. The mortality rate for patients with cancer was higher in those with poor dietary habits and malnutrition. Moreover, the tumor is capable of recovering from fasting conditions faster than normal cells, regaining its prefasting growth rate within 1 or 2 days.

Malnutrition can involve the defense mechanism in different ways. Cell-mediated immunity, which defends the body against cancer, is significantly affected. Thymus-dependent lymphocytes are markedly depressed in patients with severe malnutrition and in those with an iron deficiency. These deficiencies are subsequently reversed by nutritional repletion. Nitrogen balance was also found to affect cellular immune responses, and there is evidence that nutritional constituents modify the role of carcinogens through the activity of specific enzymes. The activities of these enzymes are depressed by protein deficiency, starvation, a fat-free diet, and certain vitamin deficiencies. Low protein levels suppress the metabolic enzymes in the liver so that the carcinogenicity of some ingested chemicals persists. Minerals must be supplied because they play an essential role in fighting cancer. Serum iron and zinc levels are reduced while copper is elevated during the active phases of cancer. Moreover, zinc is essential for protein synthesis and plays a major role in DNA and RNA synthesis. Levels of zinc and copper in serum are interrelated and affect vitamin A and retinol metabolism. A diet rich in calcium, iron, copper, zinc, selenium, and protein reduces the immunosuppressive effect of cadmium and lead. Other trace metals such as manganese and nickel also play major roles.

Body weight can be used as a yardstick and a rough measure of nutritional status. With continued weight loss, serum albumin levels will eventually drop, but it will be a late occurrence and cannot be used as a reliable early indication of poor nutritional status. The situation is different in children, where weight alone cannot be used for this purpose. Children grow fast and may even gain weight or stay at the same weight without evidence of malnutrition. A child can grow taller in a short period of time – even during a hospital stay – with an expected weight gain because of the increase in height. Weight and height should be considered together when assessing the absence or presence of malnutrition in a child [18]. Therefore, weight and height ratios are better indicators of early nutritional problems; a weight/height ratio of less than 20% is a criterion for malnutrition. Weight gain through fluid retention, edema or ascites should be monitored closely.

Cachexia in cancer patients occurs less frequently today than in the past because cancer is being detected earlier, nutritional problems are better understood, and the disease is managed better. Cachexia is mostly a late manifestation. The concept that explains the mechanism of malnutrition in cancer patients, developed in 1909, maintains that competition for nutrients between host and cancer cells is responsible. *Theologides* [49] theorized that cancer peptides throw the host's metabolism into a chaotic state by activating and inactivating enzymes and increasing the energy expended as host metabolites are trapped by the growing cancer. However, the host's basal metabolic rate is not elevated. As the tumor grows in bulk, its nutritional requirements increase until they cannot be met adequately by the body. Consequently, a larger intake of food is required, greater than the cancer patient can ingest.

Nitrogen Trap

Without a doubt, most of the nitrogen incorporated in the cancerous tumor is derived from body tissues and the metabolic pool, but not directly from food. As nitrogen flows in only one direction, it is trapped in the cancer cells, which continue to extract amino acids from body proteins. Patients with cancer will soon be in negative nitrogen balance, which gets worse as the growth and bulk of the tumor progress.

As in leukemia with its widely disseminated cancer cells, and in lymphoma, or advanced stages of cancer, the degree of negative nitrogen balance becomes worse and is paralleled by weight loss. Local excision of the tumor – or what is described as debulking the cancer – is accompanied by improvement in the patient's condition and ability to reverse the cachectic process. Although the amino acid content of tumor cells varies widely from that of normal cells, amino acid profiles in the blood of cancer patients are the same as those in normal persons. Interestingly, attempts were made to treat cancer patients by producing an amino acid deficiency. Arginine, in particular, was used to deprive the rapidly growing tumor cell of amino acid, the most essential element for its growth.

Energy Drain

As the tumor drains the body of energy, it consumes large amounts of glucose at the host's expense. Anaerobic glycolysis is the predominant process for energy production, which results, at the same time, in lactic acid formation. Cancer cells have a limited supply of oxygen because they divide rapidly and usually outgrow the available vascular supply. Consequently, the amount of oxygen available to the tumor cells diminishes, a condition described as *hypoxia,* or *anoxia* in severe cases. This energy drain and hypercatabolic state are aggravated by the recycling of lactic acid and pyruvate-forming glucose, further draining energy from normal channels. Additional weight loss follows, accompanied by fatigue. Increased lactic acid constituents can be demonstrated in patients with a massive tumor burden, according to *Gold* [22], who proposed that the inhibition of gluconeogenesis, vital to cancer cells, inhibits cancer growth. Treating cancer by depriving tumors of their essential constituents is still experimental, but results to date appear promising. Intravenous glucose-dextrose was also used to combat the lactic acidosis produced by tumor cells. The patient's metabolic build-up may be aggravated by anorexia, vomiting, diarrhea, or malabsorption. The loss of vitamins and electrolytes results in their imbalance, and fluid and electrolyte depletion may intensify. Blood loss or bone marrow suppression caused by the disease or its management adds to the worsening situation.

Nutrition as a Supportive Measure in Cancer Management

Maintaining a cancer patient in good general health requires proper and aggressive management. Nutritional equilibrium and a positive nitrogen balance are required for tissue healing. Problems of convalescence are reduced and early ambulation is possible.

Nutritional counseling should be given from the start and continued throughout treatment, as it was found to be particularly helpful for critically ill patients. Minor nutritional problems can be corrected by a mere change in eating habits, encouraging the patient to eat small frequent meals throughout the day. Different food recipes to make food more palatable or easier to swallow and which contain the required nutritional supplements, are usually useful. Moral support from family and friends and a pleasant dining atmosphere sometimes help. Weight-watching should be maintained because weight gain in patients who have lost weight is a gradual process and needs to be supervised closely. Some patients can be expected to gain weight quicker than others. Gaining or maintaining body weight is a good indicator, usually accompanied by a reasonably good prognosis. Food supplements are of benefit and may be required, but they cannot replace food. Medication for pain, for difficulty in swallowing, and for anorexia, nausea or vomiting helps to tide the patient over critical times. *Supportive mouth feeding* – through a nasogastric (N–G) tube – of highly nutritive, easily ingested and digested food with added supplements may be given to patients who have problems with swallowing, or in the presence of an obstruction to food. *Transfusion therapy,* using whole blood or selected replacement with packed red cells or platelets, may be required in cases of anemia and bleeding.

Intravenous Hyperalimentation

Intravenous fluids for hyperalimentation is the most intensive and quickest modality for achieving a positive nitrogen balance, quicker than any other form of nutritive supplementation. It is only indicated if the patient is having problems with chewing or swallowing, or is vomiting, has severe pain, or is severely depressed, abstaining from food, and has suicidal tendencies.

Historically, hyperalimentation was studied by *Dudrick* and coworkers (1968), who proved that the gastrointestinal tract is no longer necessary to provide the body with adequate nutrients [18]. Nutrients can be administered without the need for digestion by gastric, pancreatic, or biliary secretions.

A *hyperalimentation team* is specially trained to introduce catheters into central or peripheral veins and is experienced in controlling sepsis. These teams should be able to monitor different mixtures with different constituents and caloric requirements, changing them according to the patient's condition. Metabolic disturbances such as hyperchloremic acidosis and other created metabolic problems along with fluid overload may occur and should be avoided because many patients may not respond to or benefit from it.

Overweight and Cancer Incidence

Just as malnutrition has its adverse effect on cancer, so does overweight. A positive association has been reported between the higher frequency of cancer and the increased food intake with resultant increased body weight and obesity. Rats of heavier weights were noticed to be at greater risks for tumors than lighter rats; the occurrence of certain tumors was closely associated with increased levels of protein intake. In beef cattle, the incidence of spontaneous ocular carcinomas was 14% in heavier animals fed on prairie pastures and supplemented during the winter, compared with a 1.5% incidence in animals fed on poor pastures. Japanese women who emigrated to the United States were found to have a higher incidence of breast and colon cancers than those living in Japan. According to epidemiologists, this is caused by the higher fat content of food in the American diet.

High Fat Intake and Cancer

In Finland, the fat intake is high compared to that in the USA, yet Finns have a very low incidence of breast and colon cancer, indicating that other factors may be involved. Stress is among the factors suggested, as the pace of life is much quicker in the USA. However, other factors are also suspect. *Burkitt et al.* [10] found that the incidence of cancer in Connecticut is 51.8 per 100,000 population, in contrast to 3.5 per 100,000 in Uganda. In addition, 'they believe' that the increased death rate among nonwhites is definitely related to dietary, coupled with socioeconomic changes. *Burkitt's* hypothesis explains that the higher incidence of cancer of the colon is associated with a higher dietary fat content in the absence of an adequate fiber intake.

E. L. Wynder [35] and *Wynder et al.* [36] made almost the same observation and confirmed that a diet high in animal fat and protein definitely correlates with the high incidence of cancer of the colon, adding that the higher the economic class, the greater the mortality rate [58, 59]. *Burkitt* found more anaerobic bacteria in the flora of the gut of people eating a Western diet than in those on a typical Japanese or vegetarian diet. Both bile acids and the bacteria produced promoted the production of carcinogens.

Recently, the theory relating fat to carcinogenesis was given a significant boost. Both saturated and unsaturated fats are definitely implicated in the etiology of cancer of the breast and colon. Although fat in the diet is not considered a carcinogen, it appears to act as a cancer promoter, altering metabolic pathways and making tissues more susceptible to the tumorigenesis of other exogenous or endogenous factors.

Fiber Content in Diet

Plant fiber in food is an inert bulky substance that plays a major role against cancer of the gastrointestinal tract because its components may exert protective effects on the intestinal wall. Epidemiologically, *Malhortra* [33] indicated that there is a low incidence of cancer of the colon in Northern India, where the diet contains large amounts of cellulose fibers. The fiber hypothesis was widely popularized by *Burkitt* and his colleagues [10, 58]. This preventive role of fiber against cancer of the colon has gained a lot of publicity. The Western diet includes large amounts of animal fat, sugars, and proteins, highly refined cereal products; and a reduced fiber content, which are considered to be responsible for the increased incidence of cancer of the colon in Western countries. In addition, both dietary fibers and intestinal flora affect already ingested carcinogens or procarcinogens. The intra-alimentary carcinogen concentration is diluted by the bulk of the stool because of its high fiber content. Thus, the carcinogenic effect is lessened by the shorter transit time induced by the increased fiber intake. Moreover, fiber has an indirect effect on bile salts, cholesterol, and fat metabolism and alters the bacterial flora of the gut. Fiber increases the excretion of sterols and bile acids in stools, thereby reducing the enterohepatic recycling of these compounds and their possible conversion to polycyclic aromatic hydrocarbon carcinogens by the flora of the gut. On the other hand, a low fiber content prolongs the transit time of stools, prolonging the contact between gut mucosa and carcinogenic metabolites of bacteria active on bile acids.

Cancer of the colon may have more than one predisposing factor, the most salient one being increased animal fat with decreased fiber intake. Both in Argentina and in the United States cancer of the colon has the same high incidence related in both cases to the high level of beef consumption and high animal fat intake, since both are major cattle-producing countries. The per capita beef consumption in Argentina is as high as it is in the United States. Finland has a low incidence of colorectal cancer because the Finnish diet is high in fiber. In Japan, the fat intake represents 12% of the daily calories, compared to 40% in the United States, but Japanese emigrants to the United States will develop the same high incidence of cancer of the colon when they change to the dietary habits and increased fat consumption prevalent in the United States.

Also, it has been postulated that a diet deficient in vitamin A can augment the induction of colonic tumors that result from an increased amount of chemical carcinogens and an elevated tryptophan level. Some authorities have even suggested analyses of the chemical and bacterial content of feces might distinguish high-risk from low-risk populations; individuals on a high-fat diet may have different intestinal microflora and different levels of specific bacterial enzymes.

Diet and Gastric Cancer

It was noted that the death rate from carcinoma of the large bowel is inversely related to that due to gastric cancer. Dietary studies of the increased incidence of gastric cancer revealed the disease was associated with a high intake of starchs such as potato, flour, and cereals and a concurrent lower intake of fresh products. It was also speculated that gastric cancer may be related to the presence of large amounts of polycyclic hydrocarbons and nitrosamines in food. In Japan, the high intake of talc-treated rice is suspect. A high incidence of cancer of the stomach was also found in low-income groups and in those with an increased intake of smoked foods and a low intake of vitamin C. However, the incidence of stomach cancer in the United States has decreased due to the increased year-round consumption of food containing vitamin C, which antagonizes formation of putative gastric carcinogens [54].

Vitamins and Cancer

The link between cancer and vitamins is not clear. However, a vitamin deficiency or excess in animals may either enhance or inhibit the development of cancer, depending on the specific carcinogen or vitamin involved. When thiamine supplements were given to the animals, 50% developed tumors of the bladder. Conversely, vitamin C had a protective effect against gastric carcinoma due to its action on nitrosamines.

Vitamins function as coenzymes and act as cellular antioxidants responsible for cellular respiration. A deficiency or excess leads to changes in protein, nucleic acid, carbohydrates, fat, and mineral metabolisms. In 1941, *Kensler et al.* [28] found that riboflavin has a definite anticarcinogenic effect. A diet low in vitamin B complex and copper may potentiate the carcinogenic activity of the azodyes. A vitamin A deficiency was closely related to the development of tumors of the salivary gland and caused precancerous epithelial changes. Concomitantly applied, vitamin A prevented the carcinogenic effect of chemicals. Large amounts of vitamin A to Syrian hamsters protected them against cancer of the forestomach and small intestine. However, some investigators warn against the excess intake of vitamin A as some tumors may require it for their own growth. The function of IgG antibodies necessary for the defense against cancer can be impaired by a deficiency of vitamins A, C and biotin. A deficiency of vitamin B (pyridoxin, folic acid, riboflavin, pantothenic acid) would impair the entire immune system.

Detoxification of carcinogenic material is dependent on vitamin E. Its deficiency would decrease N-demethylase activity, detoxification of certain carcinogenic aromatic amines, and promote the carcinogenic transformation of 2-aminofluorine. Its presence also inhibits membrane lipid peroxidation, which is known to be carcinogenic. Large amounts of dietary α-tocopherol to C57-laden female mice reduced the yield of sarcomas without specifically identifying the exact reasons for these results.

The role of vitamin C is very controversial. It plays a key role in maintaining the intercellular matrix, whose integrity is important for the growth and proliferation of tumors. It plays also a definite role in inhibiting hyaluronidase and influences the humoral and cellular immune function. The metabolic process associated with cell repair also depends on vitamin C.

And, this vitamin was reported to inhibit the transformation progress of cancer cells beyond initiation. Vitamin C also has a definite inhibitory effect in vivo and in vitro on the nitrosation of secondary amines so that the effect of nitrosamine carcinogenesis is reduced or eliminated. Carbon tetrachloride and nitrosamines deplete body stores of ascorbic acid.

J.J. De Casse et al. [16] studied the effect of ascorbic acid on rectal polyps and found that daily supplements of 3 g may have a beneficial effect on human cancer. Conversely, a controlled study by *Cregan et al.* [13] failed to confirm the therapeutic benefit of a daily 10-gram dose of vitamin C to patients with adenocarcinoma. *Cregan* added that vitamin C can be toxic and should not be used indiscriminately. However, *Oncology Times* (vol. 3, July 1981) reported that *Linus Pauling,* the two-time Nobel laureate, has strong views on the role of vitamin C as an anticancer agent. In his defense, Dr. *Pauling* mentioned that vitamin C has a general detoxifying effect [11]. Administering it concomitantly with other anticancer drugs might require larger doses of the latter chemotherapeutic agents than if vitamin C were not given. This is why treatment failures occur, but no one had paid any attention to these facts. *Pauling* asserted that the incidence of cancer related to age is less with large doses of vitamin C; if 10 g of vitamin C are given daily, there is a 75% decrease in the incidence of cancer. He also maintains that the claim all vitamin C above the level of 150 mg is lost in the urine is incorrect because only one-sixth is lost; the remainder stays in the bowel and 50% may enter the bloodstream.

Vitamin C protects against cancer of the gastrointestinal tract and since it is excreted in the urine, it also protects against cancer of the bladder. Taken with food containing nitrites, it prevents the formation of carcinogenic nitrosamines, thus protecting against cancer of the stomach. *Pauling* himself, 80 years of age, buys 1 kg of vitamin C for $ 12.00 and takes 4–8 g in the morning in orange juice, adding baking soda to raise the acidity to a pH of 4.1. He won a research grant from the NCI after eight previous applications had been rejected.

The failure of high doses of vitamin C to benefit patients with adenocarcinomas was studied by Dr. *Cregan et al.* [13] in a randomized double-blind comparative study of daily doses of 10 g of vitamin C with a placebo. Vitamin C was not found to increase patient survival, as concluded from the nonrandomized study conducted in Vale of Levin, Scotland. Dr. *Curtis Mettlin,* Director of Cancer Control and Chief of Epidemiology at Roswell Park Memorial Institute, in his study of nutrition and cancer, related esophageal cancer to vitamin C intake and a risk reduction with vitamin A.

Vitamin Analogs

Because cancer cells require nutrients for growth and proliferation, they are susceptible to nutritional deficiencies. Vitamin analogs that interfere with the normal utilization of vitamins affect tumors. Methotrexate, which interferes with the normal cellular function of folic acid, has been useful in the treatment of cancer. Other vitamin analogs such as isoriboflavin, isopyrithiamin, and isodesoxypyridoxine are antagonists of riboflavin, pyrithiamin, and desoxypyridoxine, respectively. They are of no value in the treatment of neoplastic disease. Retinol and B retinoic analog do play a role in cancer management since they help to prevent hyperplasia and metaplasia.

Can We Prevent or Stop Cancer by Dieting?

This question has been raised recently [9–11, 14, 24, 44, 49, 50, 54]. Epidemiologists, observing the association between breast cancer and dieting, suggested it might be possible to alter the risk of breast cancer through diet. *Angelus E. Papatestas* reported to the Society of Surgical Oncology at its 33rd annual meeting in 1980 that obesity coupled with a high serum cholesterol level in patients with cancer of the breast resulted in dismal 5-years survival figures. With a decrease in serum cholesterol, studies showed an inhibitory effect on tumor cell growth. At the same time, increased cholesterol levels were associated with the increased growth rate of tumor cells. These findings support the concept of a link between diet and breast cancer.

Unfortunately, the American diet is the product of industrial innovation supported by strong advertising. Companies compete to produce a variety of goods, at the same time promoting and encouraging overeating and nonselectivity in the choice of food. The American innovation, the supermarket, displays large arrays of goods packed and presented in a very appealing manner. Social affluence and the consumer's readily available supply of money enables him to buy from an abundance of goods which, combined with an ignorance of nutritional facts, help promote overeating. Eighty million Americans are said to be overweight and the average American is considered fat.

The problem of food and cancer is not easy to solve by various restrictions, limitations, or different legislation. Despite the enforcement of laws like the Endangered Species Act that protect animals from extinction by forbidding actions that jeopardize their existence or modify their habitats, there is no similar legislation to protect humans against themselves. Good health, obviously, cannot be legislated, yet nutritional education and counseling along with changes in eating habits or lifestyles may be helpful. It is easier not to acquire a certain habit than to stop it after it has been practized for many years.

Today, the lay public has become increasingly aware of the relationship between overeating and cancer, and obesity is becoming one of the worst stigmas in the United States. Today, different food items have the exact number of calories indicated on the package, making people aware of the calories they are about to eat, and luring them to eat fewer calories every day. The market is replete with different publications and books to help people lose weight. Today, Americans consume one-third to one-half the amount of candy they consumed in 1965, according to the US Consumer and Food Economic Institute. Jogging to lose weight has become very fashionable.

Stress and the Mind – Behavioral Changes and the
Dilemma of Predisposing Factors

Stress and the Mind

Stress occurs when we are confronted with situations with which we cannot cope. The term was introduced in 1950 by *Selye* [43], the first author to write on the subject of stress. The word later became popular, and in 1958 the articles written about the subject numbered 10,000. Stress is now in-grained in our daily language and is even becoming a media event. It has surpassed the common cold as the most common public health problem and costs the nation around $ 10 to $ 20 billion annually in losses in industrial productivity. Equilibrium between the outside world and the individual can be disturbed by the sudden onset of stress. Usually body defenses can cope with stress with the help of the mind, which has the capacity to elevate the stress threshold and enhance the restoration process. The innate capabilities of different body functions are components of the 'healing way' of nature. Recently, methods have been developed to reduce the impact of stress. Self-regulation that governs the mind and the body enhance the feeling of inner strength that would be capable of creating self-directed efforts which help one to achieve self-control and feelings of self-effectiveness. Transcendental meditation, biofeedback, and other behavioral modification methods help the person to cope with stressful situations. Medications can also benefit in times of stress, and hypnosis also was found to promote life-enhancing attitudes and recovery. Faith and religious beliefs may be of great help in directing ones natural drive to restore previous nonstressful conditions. Good family relations are also known to be helpful in stressful times. Certain life stresses, such as divorce, death of a spouse, or other similar catastrophic situations, are known to increase human susceptibility to disease and were found to be common occurrences before cancer appeared. People differ in their capacity to receive and adapt to stressful disastrous situations, which are most often accompanied by a sudden change, with overwhelming physical injury and an obvious threat to life. Most cancer patients and their families live stressful lives and their mechanism for coping with stress has been inadequate and ineffective. A prospective study of medical students who developed cancer, comparing their family relations with those of other students who remained healthy [50], showed that closeness to parents was lacking in students who later developed cancer. Students who remained healthy had close relationships with their parents. Cancer was also expected in persons with certain behaviors, and psychologic counseling has been reported to avert disease, particularly in those at high risk [23, 24].

Lansky et al. [29] studied cancer coupled with parental discord and divorce in parents of 191 children treated for cancer over a 7-year period. The divorce rate was lower in this group than in other married couples of healthy children, yet marital stress was greater than in the normal group. A group of investigators reported that cancer in women, seeking biopsy of a lump in the breast, correlates significantly with a behavior pattern of suppressed anger.

Pettingale et al. [39] ran psychologic studies on patients with cancer of the lung, who were smokers and found that they were more prone to deny and repress their emotions. *Abse et al.* [1] found that patients who had cancer of the lung and smoked tended to be less assertive than smokers in general.

Behavioral Changes in Cancer Patients

Cancer patients may undergo behavioral changes as they become panicked by the sudden shocking change in their lives. They become bewildered by the new reality and most of the time react in disbelief, unable to comprehend what is happening to them. Things may appear different and their surroundings may seem to be disturbed; they become disoriented or dislocated from the present. Sometimes, in extreme situations, they may end in personal catastrophe. The family around them may feel bewildered and confused at first, and patients confronted with an overload of new information are frustrated by the ugly feeling that they cannot decide their future or plan their lives. Suddenly, they do not have a future to plan for or dream about. At the beginning of this dilemma, the variation in behavior among cancer patients is usually shaped by several factors: their ability or inability to cope with stress, family relations, cancer prognosis, socioeconomic status, age, sex as well as their philosophic beliefs and faith – all mold their particular patterns of behavior. Accompanying emotions may exaggerate these changes, a situation mimicked by the dreamer who is upset by a nightmare more frightening than reality. Likewise, cancer patients are frightened and feel helpless in this new experience. Sometimes a patient is unable to vent his feelings and outside help is indicated. Moreover, a patient's ability to conceal his behavior varies widely, and usually family and close friends help to uncover hidden problems [15, 17, 31, 38, 55].

The cancer patient's *psychologic adaptation* is dependent on ego strength. After a brief or prolonged endeavor to adapt to heavy pressure, a patient may succeed in coping well with primary problems or may end up being surrounded by an overpowering apathy and failure to adapt. The patient may end in psychologic collapse characterized by total withdrawal and a feeling of incarceration and isolation. Ego strength usually correlates positively with the patient's use of effective coping strategies, according to *Worden* [57]. Maladaptation or a delay could be remedied by outside help and psychologic support. Challenges are usually at their maximum at the time of diagnosis, but may continue to linger to variable degree during management. It is of great help to know how the patient formerly coped with stress. A suspicious person may doubt the physician's ability to cope with his problem or whether an eventual cure is possible. A dependent person will always need attention and care at the same time; an independent person may not reveal much about his condition and progress. It is reasonable to assume that the behavior of cancer patients at the end of treatment is to a great extent shaped by differences in personality.

No doubt prognosis also has its effect. Yet two successfully treated patients may not have the same attitude towards their future. One may be grateful he is out of the woods; the other may ask: why me?

Different behaviour changes may occur and should be discussed:

(1) *Fears of cancer.* Fear is an obviously overwhelming emotion, varying in its intensity and duration, and a composite of different elements.

Fear of death is the first impact of cancer. When a patient learns of his diagnosis, an immediate fear of death may occur. Recently, this perception of cancer as a sentence of death has been ameliorated somewhat by the improved survival rate. Philosophically, although death is a natural ending for us all, the thought of it is always distasteful, even to those eager to go to heaven (they still want to do that without dying).

The fear of cancer itself regardless of its outcome. Cancer is considered an insidious disease that invades the body. Since the body has no control over its spread, the end result is unpredictable. The cancer could spread, persist in spite of management, or later return. It is usually considered a disease difficult to cure.

Fear of mutilation, with loss of a breast, limb, larynx; a colostomy; or any disfigurement. The stigmata of cancer are hard to conceal from themselves or others. They remain with these people, who no longer consider themselves normal, even after complete cure.

The fear of prolonged management with stressful times and complications.

The fear of suffering, pain, sleepless nights, helplessness, and dependence on others.

The fear of sudden socioeconomic changes in life-style and the end of a decent normal life.

The intensity of fear varies with culture, society and personality even varying from one country to another, depending on advancements in technology and medical progress.

(2) *Anxiety and depression* in cancer patients usually start at the time of diagnosis and are created mostly by a head-on collision with a frightening reality. Their onset may be delayed for some time, appearing during management, or they may be transient with little or a major effect and serious consequences. According to *Peteet* [38], mismanagement may result if the patient is not given sufficient attention. The duration of anxiety and depression may vary according to personality structure, socioeconomic factors, and the seriousness of illness. During prolonged management depression may be aggravated due to the burden on both patient and family. Impending socioeconomic changes aggravate the condition. Even after treatment is complete the strain on family relations, due to lingering problems, may have a bearing on the patient's depressed condition. A prolonged state of depression may hinder the patient's ability to deal with reality. In

response to stress, fear, anxiety, and depression, reactions vary from anger to denial, distortion, sublimation, hostility, projection, frustration, and rejection; even a complete personality change may occur. *Woods et al.* [56], in a study of 49 postmastectomy patients, found that the extent of physical disability was related to the quality of life the patient led. With increased physical symptoms, there was a higher incidence of depression [56].

(3) *Denial and mental block* to the unwelcomed reality. This is a healthy sign which may vary from complete denial to slighting the situation, admitting only to the presence of a small problem or to a small tumor without ever inquiring as to whether it is benign or malignant. The patient is deeply convinced that there is no imminent problem. To distort reality may sometimes help. The patient continues to look happier and in fact uses this attitude as a shelter from reality until healthy defense mechanisms help him to adapt to the unbelievable challenge. The patient's ability to produce a mental block against cancer varies in its intensity. If denial stands in the way of realizing the need for proper management or if it compromises proper treatment, it is considered disastrous. Denial must also be distinguished from despair and complete refusal of treatment as the patient does not care whether he lives or dies. *Dansak and Cordes* [15], in their study of denial or suppression in cancer patients, stated that terminal cancer patient's reactions to death and dying may tell the hospital staff and other professionals litte or nothing about their fears or expectations – a silence construed as a defense mechanism, not denial [15]. They are not denying cancer or its consequences, but have voluntarily decided to suppress these thoughts to cope with their illness. Careful observation, they continued, would enable a physician to distinguish between denial and suppression, which is significantly different because it helps to orchestrate the needs of other patients.

(4) *Hostility and projection* of one's problems on others may sometimes occur. Using a physician, a nurse, or a technician as a scapegoat is one way of coping with distress. Unless discovered promptly and treated, hostility could aggravate management. These feelings may be evident from the start or remain dormant until they are revealed by the slightest incident. Cooperation of family and friends is required and sometimes helps.

(5) *Grief* varies among patients from those who are poor grievers to those with a deep sense of grief. Sometimes grief fluctuates between these two extremes. It usually is aggravated after surgery to remove a part of the body, particularly if the patient becomes disabled of the body image is markedly changed. Sometimes, with prolonged management, it occurs in tandem with depression.

(6) *Feeling guilt* is caused by various factors. The relation between stress and cancer makes peoples feel guilty; they may feel they were responsible for what happened to them. A patient may think he has been working too hard and not paying attention to his health. Guilt may also be related to past sins or past practices such as too much smoking or drinking. Usually a person is disturbed by the excessive anguish that he causes his family. Psychologic consultation could help eliminate such self-accusation. The patient should know and be assured that these reactions are not his alone; they also occur in others.

These different problems can be helped by assertive training and positive participation, teaching the patient how to face the challenge on his own. Patients usually respond after a time. *Weisman* [55] noticed that survival was longer in cancer patients who coped better with problems related to their disease [51].

The feeling of helplessness so common in cancer patients and the possible survival value of fighting back have led some clinicians to teach patients to fight back consciously, as suggested by *Fiore* [20]. 35 patients with breast cancer were followed and found to differ in their survival: those expressing a strong will to live did so longer than those with more timid reactions. Fighting back may be related to the patient's homeostatic mechanism. The imaginations of cancer patients may help them picture cancer cells as weak and confused, confronting the sophisticated white cells and the rest of the immunologic system. Consequently, they may improve. *Simonton and Simonton* [45] encourage and train their cancer patients to picture their tumor as overwhelmed by their bodily defenses, noting that a very powerful belief in this concept was a strong factor in the spontaneous regression of cancer seen in some patients who practice meditation.

During management, overanxiety and poor prognosis are interrelated, as noted by *Derogatis et al.* [17]. Overanxiety may be either a cause or reflection of a more active physical process, according to *Stoll* [47].

Suicide attempts are more noticeable in patients who are not undergoing treatment, particularly those with advanced disease. Gradual abstinence from food or medication is an early indication of this intention and should be handled promptly. There was no noticeable difference in the incidence of suicide attempts between males and females studied by *Louhivouri* [31]. He found that patients with a nonlocalized tumor at the time of diagnosis had a suicide risk twice that of the general population. Also, the rate was higher in patients who were undergoing palliative treatment only.

The Dilemma of Cancer: Predisposing Factors

Predisposing factors usually act as a carcinogen, a promoter of carcino-genesis, or as a procarcinogen that metabolized in the body to a carcinogen. It is not always easy to find the association between cancer and different predisposing factors. In many cases, a predisposing factor is not suspect and the fault may lie with a defective immunity – inherited or acquired – or an undetected virus. This may be the reason cancer occurs at random among the population with no apparent predisposing factor to blame. At other times, the association between cancer and predisposing causes is obvious, as with cigarette smoking and alcohol abuse, relative to cancer of the oral cavi-ties, as confirmed by different studies. The relative risk for drinkers adjusted for smoking was found to be 3.3%, 15.2%, and 10.6% for those who drink less than 6, 6–9 and 10 or more whiskey equivalents a day, respectively, as reported by *Mashberg* [34]. In the same study drinkers of 6 or more whiskey equivalents a day were found to be at a greater risk than smokers of 40 or more cigarettes a day. In addition, alcohol plays another role in cancer be-cause its dulling effect results in late presentation.

Retrospective epidemiologic studies showed that carcinoma of the up-per digestive tract is more related to alcoholic intake while carcinoma of the respiratory tract is more related to cigarette smoking [34, 60]. Recently, the rapid rise in the rate of lung cancer in women attracted everyone's attention because the Surgeon General's 1980 report focused on the health consequ-ences of their cigarette smoking [46, 52]. The increasing number of working women has also contributed to the increased incidence of cancer among them. There are many other links between cancer and certain factors, for example, vinyl chloride and cancer of the liver, radiation and leukemia, ar-senic and cancer of the skin, and many others. The multitude of predispos-ing factors are beyond containment and its is futile to try to pin down a pre-disposing factor in each case [5]. The few examples of predisposing factors previously discussed are those which have the largest impact on a wide sec-tor of the population.

References

1   Abse, D.W.; Wilkins, M.M.; Castle, R.L. van de: Personality and behavioral character-istics of lung cancer patients. J. psychosom. Res. *18:* 101–113 (1974).
2   Bailar, J.C.: Mammography: a continuing view. Ann. intern. Med. *84:* 77–84 (1976).

3   Beir, B.: The effects on populations of exposure to low levels of ionizing radiation. Com-
     mittee on the Biological Effect of Ionizing Radiations, Division of Medical Sciences, As-
     sembly of Life Sciences, National Research Council, National Academy of Sciences
     (1980).

4   Bender, M.A.: X-ray induced chromosome aberrations in mammalian cells in vivo and
     in vitro; in Buzzati-Traverso, Immediate and low level effects of ionizing radiations, pp.
     103–108 (Taylor & Francis, London 1960).

5   Berry, G.; Newhouse, M.L.: Combined effects of asbestos exposure and smoking on
     mortality from lung cancer in factory workers. Lancet *ii:* 476–479 (1972).

6   Blum, H.F.: On the mechanism of cancer induction by ultraviolet radiation. J. natn.
     Cancer Inst. *11:* 463–495 (1950).

7   Blumberg, B.S.; London, W.T.: Hepatitis B virus and primary hepatocellular cancer re-
     lationship of 'Incrons' to cancer. Viruses in naturally occurring cancer. Cold Spring Har-
     bor Laboratory Book, vol. 1 (1980).

8   Boice, J.D.; Stone, B.J.: Interaction between radiation and other breast cancer risk fac-
     tors; in Late biological effects of ionizing radiation, vol. 1, (Vienna International Atomic
     Energy Agency, 1978).

9   Burkitt, D.P.; Wright, D.H.: Burkitt's lymphoma (Livingstone, London 1970).

10   Burkitt, D.P., et al.: Effect of dietary fiber on stools and transit time and its role in the
     causation of disease. Lancet, pp. 1408–1411 (December 30, 1972).

11   Cameron, E.; Pauling, L.; Leibovitz, B.: Ascorbic acid and cancer: a review. Cancer Res.
     39: 663–681 (1979).

12   Copeland, E.M.; Dudrick, S.J.: Nutritional aspects of cancer; in Hickey, Current prob-
     lems. Cancer, vol. 1, No. 3, pp. 3–61 (Year Book Med. Publishers, Chicago 1976).

13   Cregan, E.T., et al.: Failure of high dose vitamin C (ascorbic acid) therapy to benefit pa-
     tients with advanced cancer. New Engl. J. Med. *301:* 687–690 (1979).

14   Cumbie, P.M.: Mercury levels in Georgia otter, mink and fresh water fish. Bull. env.
     Contam. Toxicol. *14:* 193 (1975).

15   Dansak, D.A.; Cordes, R.S.: Cancer denial or suppression? Int. J. Psychiat. Med. *9:*
     257–262 (1978–79).

16   De Casse, J.J., et al.: Effect of ascorbic acid in rectal polyps of patients with familial
     polyps. Surgery, St.Louis *78:* 608–612 (1975).

17   Derogatis, L.R., et al.: Psychological coping mechanisms and survival time in metastatic
     breast cancer. J. Am. med. Ass. *242:* 1504–1508 (1979).

18   Dudrick, S.J.; Wilmore, D.W.; Vars, H.M.: Long-term parenteral nutrition with growth,
     development, and positive nitrogen balance. Surgery, St.Louis *64:* 134–142 (1968).

19   Ebel, W.J.: Supersaturation of nitrogen in the Columbia River and its effect on salmon
     and steelhead trout. Fishery Bull. *68:* 1–11 (1969).

20   Fiore, N.: Fighting cancer in one patient's perspective. New Engl. J. Med. *300:* 284–289
     (1979).

21   Fraumeni, J.R., Jr. et al.: Persons at high risk of cancer. An approach to cancer etiology
     and control (Academic Press, New York 1975).

22   Gold, J.: Metabolic profiles in human solid tumors. A new technique for the utilization
     of human solid tumors in cancer research and its application to the anaerobic glycolysis
     of isologous benign and malignant colon tissues. Cancer Res. *26:* 695–705 (1966).

23   Greer, S.: Psychological enquiry: a contribution to cancer research. Psychol. Med. *9:* 81–89 (1979).

24   Greer, S.; Morris T.: Psychological attributes of women who develop breast cancer. A controlled study. J. psychosom. Res. *19:* 147–153 (1975).

25   Gunz, F.W.; Veale, A.M.O.: Leukemia in close relatives, accident or predisposition. J. natn. Cancer Inst. *42:* 517 (1969).

26   Higginson, J.: Environmental carcinogen misconception and limitations to cancer control. J. natn. Cancer Inst. *63:* 1291–1298 (1979).

27   Jose, D.G.: Undernutrition and cancer (Meet. abstr., pp. 21–22). National Cancer Week Proc. Australian Symp. on Nutrition and Cancer held in Australia, Adelaide, Australia.

28   Kensler, C.J., et al.: Partial protection of rats by riboflavin with casein against liver cancer caused by dimethylaminoazobenzene. Science *93:* 308–310 (1941).

29   Lansky, S.B., et al.: Studying childhood cancers: parental discord and divorce. Pediatrics, Springfield *62:* 184–188 (1978).

30   Larson, R.A., et al.: Chromosomal changes in hematologic malignancies. Ca-A Cancer J. *31:* No. 4 (July/August 1981).

31   Louhivouri, K.A.: Risk of suicide among cancer patients. Am. J. Epidem. *109:* 59–65 (1979).

32   Lynch, H.T.: Familial factors in bladder carcinoma. J. Urol. *122:* 458–461 (1979).

33   Malhortra, S.L.: Geographic distribution of gastrointestinal cancer in India with special reference to causation. Gut *8:* 361–372 (1967).

34   Mashberg, A.: Alcohol as primary risk factor in oral squamous carcinoma. Ca-A Cancer *31:* No. 3 (May/June 1981).

35   McKusick, V.A.; Ruddle, F.H.: The status of the gene map of the human chromosome. Science *196:* 390–405 (1977).

36   Miller, E.C.; Miller, J.A.: Mechanism of chemical carcinogens. Cancer, N.Y. *47:* 1055–1064 (1981).

37   Owerbach, D., et al.: Genetics of the large external transformation sensitive (LETS) protein: assignment of a gene coding for expression of LETS to human chromosome 8. Proc. natn. Acad. Sci. USA *75:* 5640–5644 (1978).

38   Peteet, J.R.: Depression in cancer patients – an approach to differential diagnosis and treatment. J. Am. med. Ass. *241:* 1487–1489 (1979).

39   Pettingale, K.W.; Greer, S.; Tee, D.E.: Serum Ig A and emotional expression in breast cancer patients. J. psychosom. Res. *21:* 395–399 (1977).

40   Richins, R.T., et al.: Total mercury in water, sediment and selected aquatic organism, Carson River, Nevada 1972. Pesticides Monit. J. *9:* 44 (1975).

41   Rowley, J.D.: Mapping of human chromosomal regions related to neoplasia, evidence from chromosomes 1 and 17. Proc. natn. Acad. Sci. USA *74:* 5729–5733 (1977).

42   Rugh, R.: The impact of ionizing radiation on the embryo and fetus. Am. J. Roentg. Rad. Ther. nucl. Med. 89–182–190, pp. 103–104 (1963).

43   Selye, H.: The stress of life (McGraw-Hill, New York, 1956).

44   Siegel, S.M.: Mercury: aspects of its etiology and environmental toxicity. Botanical Sci. Pap. No. 33 Hawaii University, Honolulu (1973).

45   Simonton, O.C.; Simonton, S.S.: Belief systems and management of the emotional aspects of malignancy. J. transpersonal Psychol. *7:* 29–47 (1975).

46 Stellman, S. D.: Women's occupations, smoking and cancer and other diseases. Ca-A Cancer J. *31:* No. 1 (January/February 1981).
47 Stoll, B. A.: Risk factors in breast cancer. Br. med. J. *iv:* 201–203 (1970).
48 Tannenbaum, A.: The initiation and growth of tumors – Introduction. 1. Effects of underfeeding. Am. J. Cancer *38:* 335–350 (1940).
49 Theologides, A.: Cancer cachexia. Cancer, N.Y. *43:* 2004–2012 (1979).
50 Thomas, C. B., et al.: Family attitudes reported in youth as potential predictors of cancer. Psychosom. Med. *4:* 287–302 (1979).
51 Unna, P. G.: Carcinom der Seemannshaut; in Hirschwald, Die Histopathologie der Hautkrankheiten (Springer, Berlin 1894).
52 US Department of Health and Human Services, Public Health Services: The health consequences of smoking for women. A report of the Surgeon General, p. 118 (1980).
53 Walker, A. R. P.; Burkitt, D. P.: Colonic cancer – hypothesis of causation, dietary prophylaxis and future research. Dig. Dis. *21:* 910–917 (1976).
54 Weisburger, J. H.: Mechanism of action of diet as a carcinogen. Cancer, N.Y. *43:* 1987–1995 (1979).
55 Weisman, A. D.: Coping behavior and suicide in cancer; in Cullen et al. (ed.), Cancer, the behavioral dimensions, pp. 331–358 (Raven Press, New York 1976).
56 Woods N. F., et al.: Women with cured breast cancer, a study of mastectomy patients in North Carolina. Nurs. Res. *27:* 279–285 (1978).
57 Worden, J. W.: Ego strength and psychosocial adaptation to cancer and effectiveness in resolution of problems. Psychosom. Med. *40:* 585–592 (1978).
58 Wynder, E. L.: Dietary habits and cancer epidemiology. Cancer, N.Y. *43:* 1955–1961 (1979).
59 Wynder, E. L., et al.: Environmental factors of cancer of the colon and rectum. Cancer, N.Y. *20:* 1520–1561 (1967).
60 Wynder, E. L.; Stellman, S. D.: Comparative epidemiology of tobacco related cancers. Cancer Res. *37:* 4608–4622 (1977).
61 Zuelzer, W. W.: Genetic aspects of leukemia. Semin. Hematol. *6:* 228 (1969).

Chapter 4

Race and Socioeconomic Variations in Cancer

Incidence of Cancer According to Geographic Location and Social Class

Geographic Variation

Different studies found that the problems associated with cancer vary from one country to another. Also, certain cancers are more prevalent in some areas than in others. A good example of the geographic variation of cancer is Burkitt's lymphoma, which has a characteristic distribution, in that belts of high and low incidence are found in Africa [1]. High-frequency areas are found around lakes in regions with temperatures higher than 60 °F during the winter and a rainfall exceeding 20 inches. Relatively low incidences are found in regions with altitudes above 5,000 feet.

The Epstein-Barr Virus (EBV) was found to be the most probable causative agent of Burkitt's lymphoma, and malaria is considered a predisposing factor. The EBV infection is spread mainly through saliva – by breastfeeding babies in nurseries and kissing in adults. Biting insects may also spread the disease, in which case an epidemic of Burkitt's lymphoma results.

The relationship between human leukemia and bovine lymphosarcoma and livestock population densities was noticed. Nasopharyngeal carcinoma is known to occur more frequently in East Asia; carcinoma of the bladder occurs more frequently in Egypt because of bilharziasis; liver carcinoma in certain areas of Africa; and breast and colon carcinoma in Western societies. In Northern China, there is a noticeable high incidence of poultry and human esophageal carcinoma [2], the third most frequent neoplasia in humans following breast and cervical cancers. In Linhsien county of Honan Province, esophageal cancer was the leading cause of mortality. In that province, nitrosamines and their precursors were found in pickled vegetables, while a candidum fungus was isolated from pickles. Both are known to provoke an epithelial hyperplasia before the malignancy develops. These changes were particularly noticeable with vitamin C deficiencies. In Japan and in Central Europe, Finland, Iceland, West Germany and part of the USSR, the incidence of stomach cancer is high.

No one common factor accounts for a particular geographic distribution. Only gastric cancer was more noticeable in agricultural provinces and may be related to the nitrite fertilizers and the nitrosamines used as preservatives. Some local habits are: heating fats and smoking mutton increases their content of polycyclic hydrocarbons, which are associated with a high incidence of cancer. The familial aggregations noted may be due to occupational or socioeconomic factors. Pancreatic cancer has a high incidence in Japan, but generally has an urban preponderance. It is always known as a disease of the city, compared to gastric carcinoma, which has a rural preponderance. In the USA, breast cancer accounts for one-tenth of all breast cancers diagnosed worldwide, with Canada having the same incidence. Colorectal cancer occurs with a high incidence in both the USA and Europe, accounting for 15% of all newly diagnosed cancers in white women, slightly less in white men, and even less in blacks. While the incidence is 38.6 per 100,000 population per year in the USA, it is 1.3 per 100,000 population per year in Nigeria. There is an inverse relationship between the incidence of cancer of the stomach and colorectal cancer; countries with a high rate of stomach cancer tend to have a low rate of colorectal cancer. Moreover, there is a distinct social class with a higher incidence of colorectal cancers.

Studies of the lowest incidences of cancer in different geographic locations and social classes are worth mentioning. Cancers of the lung, colon, uterus, and kidney are lowest in Uganda, Nigeria and among blacks of South Africa. Cancers of the pancreas, urinary bladder, and breasts are lowest in Singapore. Hepatocellular cancer is lower in the United States than in Mozambique and among South African blacks. Nutritional factors may play a major role in this low incidence rate.

Social Class and Cancer

Cancer of the cervix occurs most often among the poor and low socioeconomic classes. Its incidence usually declines with improved standards of living. Conversely, lymphomas are more prevalent among prosperous segments of society. And, demonstrated disease aggregates in Hodgkin's disease may be related to environment or unproved infectious elements, but need further study. Head and neck cancer, particularly esophageal cancer, correlate more frequently with poor dentition and oral hygiene and with the excessive consumption of alcohol and smoking habits.

Change of Cancer Incidence

Immigrants usually show changes in their incidence of cancer, adjusting to the incidence rates in areas to which they immigrate. Japanese women who have immigrated to the USA acquire the incidence rate of breast cancer for women in the USA. The same applies to colon and stomach cancers. Apparently, the socioeconomic habits and environmental factors affect the incidence of cancer more than racial difference. For example, the incidence of cancer of the lung is increasing among females as they acquire a greater smoking habit [3]. Conversely, the incidence of cancer of the stomach has declined more steeply in whites than in blacks but the average mortality rate remains higher in black males than in white males due to the decreased number of high-risk white persons from foreign countries, who have immigrated to the USA. The decreased incidence is also attributable to eating less smoked meat. Another version is that a greater proportion of blacks live in urban areas; accordingly, the incidence of stomach cancer is expected to be higher in black males. Dr. *Jack E. White,* Director of Harvard University Cancer Research, emphasized that cancer in blacks is usually diagnosed at a later stage, which hopefully will change as their standard of living and socioeconomic status improve. At the same time, black females have exhibited a lower incidence of cancer than white males and females, due to the same socioeconomic variations.

The incidence of pancreatic cancer is rising at the rate of 15% per decade. The increased intake of fat and cholesterol is suspected to be the cause; and increased cigarette smoking may be an additional underlying cause. Diabetes, on the other hand, is associated with a twofold increase in the incidence of pancreatic cancer, particularly among cigarette smokers and heavy consumers of alcohol.

There is an inverse relationship between gastric and pancreatic cancer. In the USA the decrease noted in gastric cancer was accompanied by a rise in pancreatic cancer.

First-generation immigrants from areas with high rates of stomach cancer and low rates of colorectal cancer tend to retain part of the previous trend – with a continued increased incidence of cancer of the stomach, and a concurrent high colorectal cancer risk. In metropolitan Toledo there was a 66% reduction in the average annual age-adjusted incidence of cervical squamous cell carcinoma and a 61% reduction in death rate when the periods from 1935 to 1938 and 1971 to 1974 were compared. These reductions were mainly due to screening and the use of the Pap test. The decrease for both morbidity and mortality, however, was not pronounced in women 50 years of age or younger. The reduction in death rate was not pronounced in black females.

References

1   Burkitt, D. P.; Wright, D. H.: Burkitt's lymphoma (Livingstone, London 1970).
2   Ha Hsien-Wen: Esophageal carcinoma in Northern China. Oncology Times *3:* No. 2 (February 1981).
3   Stillman, S. D.: Women's occupations, smoking and cancer and other diseases. Ca-A Cancer J. *31:* No. 1 (January/February 1981).

Chapter 5

Sexuality and Self-Esteem in Cancer

Sexuality may be directly or indirectly affected by cancer. Cancer primarily affecting the sex organs may have a serious impact on those individuals who feel the disease is a direct insult to their sexuality and their lives are now meaningless. A clear example is the occasional female with an affected breast or the male with penile carcinoma. Women and men afflicted with these problems may suffer from a hurt pride more than anything else. This may cause them to hide, concealing their disease from others. By the time they present for medical help, their disease is usually advanced. A feeling of deep humiliation is the reason for their incarceration for a long time until the problem becomes too great to bear or conceal further. Only when a foul odor becomes unbearable, or pain is severe, or there is uncontrolled bleeding, does the patient start to look for help. These are rare examples, however.

Most of the time, the person's sex life may be indirectly affected by cancer. Early in the course of the disease, sexual activity is sharply curtailed and this continues during management. Needless to say, sexuality does not flourish in a medium of depression and distress, since sex and depression are known to be antagonists. A vicious cycle may start as sex problems increase depression. Distressing emotional problems and delayed readjustments may decrease self-gratification, further dissuading both partners. As distress escalates, sexuality continues to be suppressed. In some cases the sexual dysfunction may be psychogenic, relieved after about 6 months with assistance, encouragement, and education of the remaining sexual potentials. Unfortunately, discussions of sexual matters are scarcely approached. Physicians and patients usually shy away from the problem, failing to realize that this is part of the patient's total needs. It may be that a patient is drowned in his fears, with depression making him abstain from discussing what he considers unimportant issues. Unfortunately, a patient may think it inappropriate to inquire about sex at these difficult times. Even the patient's partner is usually hesitant to ask about sex with a feeling of sympathy and fear of loss of partnership. It may never occur to the physician that the emotional or psychological needs of the patient may be boosted by solving sexual problems. Usually, the physician is hesitant and may feel that the patient's feelings might be hurt if sexual matters are discussed prematurely. Questions about sex usually vary according to age, marital status, partners, personal characteristics and closeness. Immediately after management, the questions usually asked are about resumption of sexual activity. When the patient regains confidence and hopes are renewed, partners start to put together the wreckage remaining after the storm has passed. Once they begin to think about resuming their normal lives, partners tend to ask questions about sex, particularly if encouraged by obvious improvement, and certainly in the presence of a friendly physician. Later, the questions may be about having children.

The problems of 'Body Image, Sexuality, and Self-Esteem in Cancer Patients' were discussed in 1979 at a well-attended conference in San Francisco. One of the questions discussed was: Why are sexual matters not routinely discussed from the start at the time treatment is planned? An obvious deficiency in the doctor-patient relationship was considered. There is an obvious need to legitimize the concern for sexual problems without fear or hesitation in cancer patient-physician relationships. Sexual dysfunction associated with cancer may have a bearing on the total outcome, as it might aggravate personal relationships with resulting psychologic problems. Sexuality may be affected in different forms: physical pleasure disturbance, loss of productive capacity with cessation of menstruation, loss of sexual organs or due to the mutagenic effect of management.

A decrease in sexual satisfaction is most disturbing and may be related either to organic or emotional factors, as when a patient's self-image is remarkably affected following *heroic* surgery in the head and neck area, as in the Commando procedure, or in laryngectomies, mastectomies or penile resection. The patient's potency may be hurt either by surgery, radiotherapy or chemotherapy. Colostomy patients usually have problems that are reflected on both partners, with a resulting loss of libido. Between anger and depression, 20% of women who had mastectomies were unable to look at the surgical area for an average of 22 months. They may have been afraid to face reality or were endeavoring to maintain their prior self-image. In fact, some women fear mastectomies more than the cancer itself, and a complex of *half-woman* may begin to evolve. A feeling of loss of femininity or of being no longer physically attractive is very upsetting to both sexes and may lead to psychologic regression. A woman may start dressing in a dark room or in the bathroom to avoid the watchful looks of sympathy or surprise in her husband's eyes, or any reactions different from those experienced before surgery. Obviously, there is a noticeable relationship between the intensity and frequency of symptoms and the degree of depression and resultant loss of sexual desire. Inconvenient symptoms, such as vaginal discharge, bleeding, pain or soreness in the pelvic area obviously inhibit resumption of normal sexual relationships.

These different problems may be exaggerated and further complicate the life of a single woman, a divorcee, or an unhappily married woman. These patients readily fall prey to feelings of lessened self-worth. Even well-adjusted and stabile women are not entirely protected from these feelings, but it may have a lesser impact on them. Great help could definitely be provided by a loving and understanding partner; a relationship particularly noticeable in close families. Emotional reactions are also related to age, marital status, and feelings of security. The female's attitude of being a sex symbol may greatly shape the outcome. Most women suffer greatly if they are not properly prepared for this kind of experience preoperatively as reported by *Woods and Earp* [2]. The life of a cancer patient can be made dismal by these unexpected sexual changes. A different mental outlook usually prevails for a person facing a new and unexpected challenge. The choice of prostheses and differently fitting clothes are emotionally demanding burdens on the patient's psychologic well-being. Emotional distress peaks 3 months after mastectomy, a time just before the patient resumes her normal activities and assumes her normal responsibilities according to *Worden and Weisman* [3]. Usually at these times, hopes are renewed and a person starts to worry about the future, expressing doubts about further survival, talking about her worries, and questioning herself and others about her prognosis. Early discussions of sexual problems would prepare partners emotionally and physically to adapt to a new life. Both partners should be included in the discussions from the start; stability and satisfaction can be a valued product of such intervention because later explanations, when the problem exists and depression and worries prevail, may be less convincing. If both partners are not prepared to face these critical challenges, the new experience might shatter a fragile relationship between uncaring partners. Guidance, psychotherapy, counseling, and marital sex therapy may help. Sharing a bed or sleeping in separate beds or different rooms may be alternatives, particularly for patients with excretory conduits. Sometimes, it is wise to leave the problems to be discussed and worked out, without embarrassment, to a time when both are properly prepared and made aware of the different aspects of the problem.

Many questions about living together, such as – Is cancer transmitted through intercourse or just living together under one roof? – will have to be answered. The answers may relieve many people. During prolonged radiotherapy or chemotherapy, questions about whether a person may become radioactive, whether chemicals will affect a partner, or other fears that never happen, may arise and should be properly explained. Sometimes, the simultaneous or sequential occurrence of cancer in husband and wife develops. It is usually adenocarcinomatous in nature and may be related to socioeconomic factors or some unknown reason. Most of the time sexual activity is encouraged, but the question of pregnancy while the patient is still in treatment, or later on, should be openly discussed and properly planned as the consequences on the disease and on the child may be serious. Decisions as to whether to have children should be discussed and explained. A frank discussion of comfortable positions for intercourse, for patients with different problems, might solve what might seem to be an impossible situation to the partners. Usually, early resumption of intercourse prevents the vagina from narrowing. A cream to combat dryness and digital separation of adhesions or the use of vaginal dilators are advisable until sexual intercourse can be resumed without pain. A loving, sensitive partner is of great help at these times; affection, physical love and other coital equivalence can replace vaginal coitus if sexual intercourse decreases. The desire for other physical contact may be increased since strong affections still exist, mitigating problems of sexual intercourse. Plastic surgery of the vagina, breast, or other area should be done only after a waiting period, to be sure the risk that cancer will recur is minimal.

Orgasm can be directly affected by management modalities and their complications, or by the disease itself. Cancer of the prostate, bilateral excision of the testicles, or hormonal therapy might lead to impotence. Associated psychosexual problems due to stress or profound weakness may also be closely related. Pretreatment sexual status and associated problems such as diabetes and vascular disease also have a bearing on outcome. If the neurovascular supply of the accessory sex organs is resected, potency will be affected, for example, as in the bilateral para-aortic node dissection for the management of testicular tumors. The pudendal arteries, if affected, may hinder the erectile mechanism. Sympathetic and parasympathetic nerves, if sacrificed, may affect ejaculation. Tumors of the spinal cord can also cause impotence. With complete cord transection, erection can be established by local stimulation, but it may not be voluntary, and orgasm and ejaculation rarely occur. Prolonged radiation therapy may have immediate or latent desexualizing effects. Radiation and chemotherapy as well as surgery can affect the reproductive system and at times destroy Sertoli cells responsible for effective spermatogenesis. Genetic mutagenesis may result if the germ epithelium is affected.

The azospermia induced by radiation may last for several months, but the sperm count usually returns to pretreatment levels within 3–4 years after radiation therapy is completed. Birth defects are not expected to occur after the sperm count returns to normal. Fertility is usually affected by the decreased sperm count. But sexual potency can be preserved in a high percentage of patients by the proper choice of treatment. Radiotherapy, an alternative to surgery for cancer of the prostate, does not affect potency as markedly and also results in good survival rates, according to *Harry* [1].

Sperm banks to store and preserve human sperm can be particularly important in the treatment of young people with malignancy who are looking forward to fathering children. As early as 1886, *Montezza* suggested that soldiers going to the battlefield could have their sperm frozen and still beget children as their legal heirs if they died. Successful conception and normal births after insemination with frozen sperm was reported in 1963. Through animal husbandry millions of cattle have been bred regularly from frozen sperm without an increase in congenital abnormalities. Human sperm can be stored for up to 10 years; some sperm have even been stored for over 19 years. Of 520 children born after insemination with frozen sperm, only 1% had congenital abnormalities and 8% were spontaneously aborted. In California, one of the most enlightened statutes in the USA was enacted in 1969. It confirmed that a child born as a result of conception through artificial insemination, with written consent of the husband, is legitimate offspring if the birth occurs during marriage or within 300 days after it is dissolved.

References

1   Harry, H.: Preservation of sexual potency in prostatic cancer patients after pelvic lymphadenopathy and retropubic 125 I implantation. J. Urol. *121:* 621–623 (1979).
2   Woods, N.F.; Earp, J.A.: Women with cured breast cancer. A study of mastectomy patients in North Carolina. Nurs. Res. *27:* 279–285 (1978).
3   Worden, J.W.; Weisman, A.D.: The fallacy in post mastectomy depression. Am. J. med. Sci. *273:* 169–173 (1977).

Chapter 6

Objectives of the Drive to Control Cancer

As a large number of us are in the same predicament with regard to the risk of developing cancer, we should all be concerned with the problem. To accept the status quo is a risky gamble that threatens all of our lives. Yet, it is hard to believe that there is an easy solution to this problem. No one can deny progress, however modest it may be, as there are undoubtedly subtle indications of improvement in the understanding and management of the cancer problem. Furthermore, we should be honest with ourselves and recognize more achievable objectives. For example: are we just trying to prolong the lives of cancer patients? Or are we aspiring to live in a world without cancer? Are we determined to decide the nature of our environment for ourselves and for our children? Some even claim that we are becoming a nation of 230 million guinea pigs. Many believe that the FDA is not spelling out facts about the harmful effects of different hazards we are exposed to in our everyday lives. These questions need to be answered honestly and it is time to start putting together a solid base for coherent long-term policies for ourselves and for future generations if we are to achieve meaningful goals with maximum benefits. Issues as well as objectives should be clear even though the final solution to the problem still remains in the future. The harmful effects of shortsighted policies, which are mostly reflex in nature, should be recognized as they lead to deadlocks, frustration, and despair. Our goal should be to one day achieve one if not all of the following objectives:

(1) *Cancer prevention* to eliminate all predisposing factors.

(2) *Cancer prophylaxis* in which immunodeficiencies are detected and subsequently corrected in time to prevent or inhibit carcinogenesis.

(3) *Increase the cure rate* through (a) the best use of available facilities; (b) early recognition of disease and prompt treatment; (c) discovering and using more potent methods of treatment with safe therapeutic ratios to maximize their effects on cancer cells and decrease the incidence of morbidity. Nothing would be more rewarding than a complete cure for the entire problem.

Prevention

The marked increase in the incidence of cancer in the United States and the Western world is closely related to industrialization and modernization, with an unprecedented and remarkable sophistication in life-style. What characterizes this space age are the hundreds of innovations and changes that succeeded each other in a very short period of time: new drugs, synthetics in textile and domestic uses, and cosmetics are just a few of the new changes used daily by millions of people. There is an obvious increase in X-ray exposure for various reasons; thousands are exposed, during air flights, to cosmic radiation and the higher concentration of plutonium in the compressed air of cabins, particularly during supersonic flights. The exposure is so great that air-flight attendants are advised not to fly during early pregnancy because damage to the fetus is possible from cosmic radiation and solar flares as well as radioactive freight. From the Arctic to the Antarctic, 5,000 Ci (curies) of radioactive particulates are still suspended in the air. Ozone is another hazard at high altitudes as it has radiomimetic characteristics that can produce chromosomal aberrations. Obviously, our lives seem to be infiltrated with a multitude of changes difficult to contain or define. It is equally impractical to return to the life-style of the 19th century or earlier. We cannot even eliminate the fact that the pace of life with its stresses is related to this problem. One-tenth of all cases of cancer of the breast in the world occurs in the USA. The highest incidence of colonic cancer is reported in Western societies. Lung cancer is increased worldwide more than 20 times from 1930 to 1973.

The objective of total elimination of all predisposing factors with a potential carcinogenic effect is a theoretical assumption and a dream. Although comforting to many, it is obviously hard to achieve. At present, there is no indication that we can achieve this objective. The NCI spends 15% of its budget on cancer prevention. A gradual improvement in the problem with containment from further growth starts with the enumeration of most of the hazards. Their allowable safe concentrations should be studied in different locations, and methods to determine the extent to which a person is exposed to these hazards are becoming more available through the use of small portable gadgets, worn or carried by individuals, to record the extent of exposure. A limit should be established beyond which a person is not permitted further exposure. Certainly, total elimination of these hazards is the best solution, and safer alternatives should be investigated.

The entire population is not exposed equally to these hazards. Alleys of cancer detected by an increased mortality rate from the disease are known. It is essential to realize that the shower of different carcinogens and mutagens and their interaction gradually and unnoticeably produce defects in our bodily defenses, which make us an easy prey to carcinogenesis. We tend to blame only a few of these carcinogens and contain ourselves in a small sphere, disregarding or denying the rest of the complex problem. It is ridiculous to assume that a single legislative act will solve this huge, mounting problem that has been neglected for 50 years.

New modalities, capable of detecting carcinogens and their metabolites as well as DNA-bound products in human tissues and biologic fluids, were recently introduced. These techniques are capable of providing *on-line* monitors of carcinogen exposure, as suggested by Dr. *Bernard Weinstein* [2]. Detailed knowledge of the enzyme system involved in the metabolic activation and deactivation of many chemicals is providing important tools for the recognition of a potential carcinogen so that further exposure can be reduced before it is too late. At present, detecting and monitoring different carcinogens is the only effective available way in which we can shield ourselves from this continuous shower of insults by mutagens and carcinogens in the air we breathe, the water we drink, and the food we eat.

Conflict between Health and Economy

Cleaning the environment and containing different hazards within safe limits is a complicated issue with political and financial implications. In certain locations, strict enforcement of industrial regulations has been estimated to cost as much as $ 140,000 per worker. The cost of removing all previously installed asbestos from schools and other locations has been estimated to be more than $ 330 million. The money needed to clean up all dumping sites in the country amounts to $ 40 billion.

The risk-benefit analysis is a forceful new concept. Moreover, any hasty decision may have serious economic implications that may affect thousands of people. To dismiss the problem of environmental pollution as unrelated to the cancer problem, or practically impossible to deal with, has grave consequences and ultimately may end in a catastrophe. Licensing any new industry that has no disposal and dumping system must be strictly limited in the future; regulations for industry should not be imposed but rather worked out mutually between industry and government. Working as adversaries would only delay any feasible solution and further complicate matters. In Japan, industry and government work together harmoniously for the good of all. Certainly, the good of the people should be put above all other interests. Meanwhile, the role of different agencies must continue probing and monitoring health standards.

The new social and personal styles of life play a role in the cancer problem. To blame industry and industrialization alone for the increased incidence of cancer is unfair. No doubt, people themselves contribute to the problem. For example, using public transportation rather than private cars would decrease the amount of toxic car fumes to insure cleaner and healthier air. Sacrifices should be offered on behalf of the people, and at the same time government should provide better facilities. Obviously, we are leading more sophisticated lifestyles, different from that of our ancestors. The habitual use of drugs, tranquilizers, sleeping pills, vitamins, enzymes, and hormones are just a few of the obvious differences. In an affluent society, the stresses of life, excessive smoking, sexual promiscuity, alcohol abuse and poor nutritional education with overeating habits, all add up and represent extra hazards. Clearly, cancer prevention is complicated and it will take a long time to find a solution, even with the cooperation of all involved.

Cancer Prophylaxis

Confronted with all of the frustrations of cancer prevention, the most feasible alternative is prophylaxis, since it carries with it a gleam of hope. The idea is to prepare the individual physically and mentally against the shower of insults and carcinogens that decreases the body's resistance to cancer. To increase the body's resistance and to promote early detection of any weakness in the body's defenses – inherited or acquired – should be promptly remedied, and the person watched closely for the earliest sign of the disease.

Immunologic deficiency also needs to be monitored. Familial genetic surveys are important as 160 gene traits have been linked to tumor development in man. Even unaffected family members may be gene carriers and may have offspring who can be considered at high risk for cancer.

Clinical research is also being conducted to identify cancer promoters and cancer inhibitors with the objective of potentiating inhibitors so that carcinogenesis can be aborted at its inception. Another objective is to stimulate detoxification responses with agents that block enzyme activation by carcinogens.

Chemoprevention is currently being investigated by different methods:

(1) *Retinoids,* which include natural and synthetic vitamin A, have been experimentally shown to be effective cancer-preventative agents. Their promise, in cancer prevention, involves their use during latent periods to suppress or delay the malignant process after cancer has been initiated. We must realize that their effect stops being useful once the cancer becomes invasive.

At present, preventive effects pertain only to carcinomas that arise from epithelial tissues. Retinoids are neither cytotoxic nor mutagenic but usually control cell differentiation in epithelial tissues. Natural retinoids are of limited use in the chemoprevention of cancer because their tissue distribution is inadequate and they are excessively toxic. The synthetic retinoids are more potent cancer preventatives in animals, and less toxic. A Phase I study, conducted by the National Bladder Collaborate Group A, involving individuals at high risk for bladder cancer, is in progress using 13-*cis*-retinoic acid. However, the indiscriminate use of retinoids in cancer therapy is not advisable.

Some tumors may benefit from an excess of vitamin A as they are known to be sensitive to retinoic acid, depending entirely on the quality of binding protein within the tumor. Some even suggest that the tumor should first be evaluated for its protein binding content to determine the ability of retinol analogs and of retinoic acid to combine with proteins; in this way sensitivity of the tumor can be evaluated and the value of such management assessed.

Vitamin A has been given to workers who are constantly exposed to asbestos. The retinoid analogs were used so as to prevent hyperplasia and squamous metaplasia of tracheal cells. A wide variety of compounds that inhibit carcinogen-induced neoplasm and potentiate the activity of cancer-deactivating enzymes, thus blocking the activity of chemical carcinogens in the body, are available to inhibit neoplasia of the large bowel. These are currently being investigated.

(2) *Vitamin C and α-tocopherol* are other agents that can be used for chemoprevention, because they inhibit cell transformation beyond cancer initiation and therefore have a probable role in chemoprevention, according to Dr. *William Benedict,* Associate Professor of Pediatrics at the University of Southern California [1].

Natural food constituents in vegetables such as cabbage and sprouts contain *ascorbic acid and α-tocopherol,* which also act as blocking agents to prevent carcinogens from reaching or reacting with critical target sites in the body. At times the interaction is interference with the response of cells to carcinogenic materials. The effect of blocking agents occurs most often before invasive cancer develops. After the onset of invasiveness the effect of ascorbic acid is debatable. The curative effects of ascorbic acid in the treatment of cancer have been studied in Scotland and at the Mayo Clinic. Both vitamin C and α-tocopherol have been shown to inhibit the formation of carcinogenic nitrosamines and nitrosamides, highly involved in gastric cancer. A negative association was found between the incidence of gastric cancer and the consumption of fresh fruits and vegetables containing ascorbic acids. In clinical studies the addition of fiber to ascorbic acid and α-tocopherol to the diet affected the level of mutagens in the large bowel.

(3) *Protease inhibitors* to block tumor promoters that stimulate the production of protease enzymes are commonly found in the body and may be involved in carcinogenesis. These ingredients inhibit the action of proteases, an effect promoted by diets high in vegetables and low in meat.

(4) *Vaccines* are now being tested at the NCI of Canada for their prophylactic effectiveness against lung cancer. The antigen of lung cancer is being administered to men who are at high risk of developing the disease.

(5) *The role of prophylactic surgery* in curing precancerous conditions of the skin, colonic polyps, or uterine cervix with evidence of advanced metaplasia is known to abort the carcinogenic process. Yet, prophylactic surgery varies according to the situation involved. Alveolar carcinoma of the breast is not managed in a manner similar to that for epithelial carcinoma of the ovaries because chances of bilateral involvement are not as high in carcinoma of the breast. In ovarian carcinoma, it is acceptable to resect the contralateral ovary because the chances that it is also involved are as great as the risk that its discovery will be delayed, because it is a deep-seated organ. In ulcerative colitis and familial polyposis, prophylactic colectomy has been practiced to minimize the probability of malignancy. But prophylactic removal of the opposite breast in alveolar carcinoma is an unnecessary, unacceptable procedure for two main reasons: the chances that the opposite breast will become involved are much less than in previous examples, and close follow-up as well as clinical examination can detect an early malignancy in the opposite breast.

A mirror-image biopsy is therefore justified and is an acceptable procedure in the management of the opposite, uninvolved breast.

Increased Curability

This would entail the following:

(1) Increased effectiveness of available treatment modalities.

(2) The probable discovery of treatments with specific preferential lethal effects on cancer cells, sparing normal cells.

(3) Early discovery of asymptomatic disease in its preclinical phase through probable biochemical changes or specific tumor markers that are simple, reliable, and specific enough to be dependable. Recently, the Chinese have developed some techniques using the α-proteins to discover early tumors of the liver.

(4) A broader definition and discovery of high-risk patients through routine screening and close follow-up.

(5) It is essential to provide proper information about cancer, a topic that will be discussed in the following paragraphs.

Lay Education

One in every four persons in the United States may develop cancer once in his lifetime, and deaths from cancer over the last 30 years have doubled along with a remarkable increase in cancer incidence. Yet, there has been no matching public education. People do not seem anxious to learn about cancer. They are either confused or unable to understand different facts about the disease. The fear of cancer is unparalleled by any similar feeling about any other disease or catastrophic situation, such as war. The word cancer is still taboo, and sometimes even professionals try to avoid it because of a deep-rooted fear of the disease within everyone. It is obvious that the general population's knowledge about cancer is lacking and whatever little they know is most often unclear and distorted.

Public education is urgently needed to create a clearer image of cancer. Special attention must be given to high-risk individuals and those in low socioeconomic classes, because poor people are sometimes helpless, do not seem to seek early medical advice, and tend to neglect themselves either because they are not aware of the problem or are financially unable to. Lay education is a tremendous undertaking and needs the participation of different organizations, including universities, to provide a dynamic, well-focused program that delivers essential knowledge to all. Funds for public education should be raised. Whatever education is given to the laity, does not substitute for the continued guidance of experts. The main objective is to teach people to recognize the early signs and symptoms of cancer, to eliminate the fear of this disease, and to dismiss the old concept that cancer is a death sentence. It is equally important to motivate people towards positive participation in their management. Most important, people must be taught to avoid predisposing factors or minimize their exposure to them and to seek advice, particularly if they are categorized as a 'high risk'. Everyone should listen to the news about cancer and not shy away from it. Possibly, some knowledge of the statistics might encourage people to develop a more positive attitude towards the disease. They should know that skin cancer is curable in almost 100% of cases; in Texas skin cancer is a way of life. People should also be taught that much has been learned about cancer, particularly in the last century. It is encouraging to know that an NCI-sponsored national study showed that the general public's awareness of current facts about cancer, particularly that of the female population, has increased substantially since 1973. For example, greater numbers of women are practicing breast self-examination (BSE). However, much more needs to be done to increase the percentage of women who practice BSE regularly and properly from the current 20%. The important benefits of educating the public are: it would yield more successful screening programs and a more knowledgeable, informed public.

The lay public should be familiar with the following different *warning signs of cancer:* (1) any change in bowel movement habits; (2) prolonged sore throat; (3) unusual bleeding or discharge; (4) lumps; (5) prolonged indigestion, difficulty in swallowing, unexplained weight loss; (6) recent change in a mole or wart; (7) prolonged cough or hoarseness. – Sometimes, there are unusual presentations, such as easy tiredness, anemia, occult blood and even nail brittleness, rheumatic pain or an itchy skin.

The News Media

Newspapermen look at medical news, particularly that about cancer, in the same way they do politics, economics, or sports, and report it the same way. In trying to sell their newspapers, they overlook the harm they can inflict on the uninformed public. Editing might even distort the issues further in an effort to make a good story, more interesting to readers, with the media arguing that the public has 'the right to know'. News about cancer is never weighed for its impact on the public. Specialized media writers, instead of lay reporters, may handle the news about cancer differently in newspapers, on radio or television. However, producers of the news media know that news about medical subjects attracts a large number of readers, promoting sales of their newspapers or a wider audience for their television or radio news. Moreover, the blinding competition between different news media makes them resort to flashy news items and sometimes frightening headlines. As a result, newswriters and television scriptwriters with science backgrounds are desperately needed. Unfortunately, irresponsible journalism prefers sensationalism which usually sells far better than authentic consumer education. Sometimes, the media's mass indictment of the medical profession makes coping with the situation impossible. Misinforming the public fosters mistrust and belief in the treating physician. Different publications, books, or movies usually dramatize a story with heroic prolonged suffering to make a better and more marketable story. Unfortunately, nothing about cancer cure that does not make a good story or a good movie is reported. It is equally important to report as newsworthy updated statistics about improved survival using only data from scientific reports. New modalities or machines should also be publicized. Premature announcements about different reports have an emotional impact on the public. They should not be released to the news media until further studies are properly introduced and confirmed by the medical profession. Even scientific authorities sometimes report their studies to the public prematurely. One such report from the National Academy of Science – the Supreme Court of Science – on fat intake was greeted with surprise and resentment by other scientific organizations, creating loud arguments that confused the general public and other diet-conscious people.

Interferon is not approved as a commercial product by the FDA as yet and, therefore, is still considered an experimental drug. Nevertheless, it is a classic example of how a mass of premature reports could affect the general public, especially the cancer patient. According to *Serena Stockwell (Oncology Times,* vol. 4, April 1982), interferon is being sold illegally by capable physicians to cancer patients in the United States for use outside limited clinical trials. This drug, which has an inherent toxicity of its own, was reported to contain other toxic substances, so that in unskilled hands its present use can be life-threatening, according to an Alert issued by the American Cancer Society. A black market has already been created in which the price of interferon has reached up to $ 5,000 per month per patient. Its cost may be as high as $ 60,000 or even $ 90,000 in West Germany, Mexico, and Italy. There are even reports that interferon is being sold in some health food stores and regular lectures are being given to patients on how to make 'your own interferon'. There seems to be a ready market for almost every improved method of treatment, as organized groups are formed almost instantaneously and ready to promote it. Such a situation, once created, is very difficult to combat. It is much easier to abort efforts to create this situation than to fight it once it has been established.

Sometimes certain terms stir the emotions. For example, the word victim is often used in connection with cancer but is less often used with such illnesses as coronary disease or vascular stroke where only 60% of patients survive the 1st year, a survival rate comparable only to aggressive types of cancer. Moreover, most patients who have had a stroke may never again be active in life.

Professional Education

The medical profession shares in the responsibility for public education, designed to increase their understanding of critical medical issues. It is the physician's responsibility to change the blind fear of cancer. Unfortunately, a pessimistic attitude prevails – even among members of the medical profession –, due mainly to poor and fragmented instruction about cancer at various medical schools. Updated knowledge about the management of cancer is not provided, current statistics are not available, and multidisciplinary approaches are not reflected in the programs offered. Moreover, cancer is placed at the end of the list of diseases covered and is pictured as having the worst possible prognosis. Physicians usually graduate with a poor and distorted knowledge of the disease and a pessimistic attitude about its prognosis, which they impart to the public. Even in their training, they are not adequately exposed to all of the different specialities involved in the management of cancer.

Propagation of Accurate Knowledge – Centers of Information

Death certificates are no longer the only source of information about cancer. Tumor registries have been developed where more data can be obtained. At the present time, centers of information are available where an abundance of already crystallized information is available to everyone for different uses. 800 h of information about cancer research and projects are available each month in *Cancer Line,* and this information can be provided to 1,000 locations in the United States and around the world from a computer base located at the National Library of Medicine in Bethesda, Md. Three different data bases – *Cancer Lit, Cancer Proj* and *Clin Prot* – comprise the *Cancer Line* computer system, and all are part of the International Cancer Research Data Bank. The ICRDB program was developed as a requirement of the National Cancer Act and is responsible for disseminating information about cancer research to scientists and clinicians around the world.

Cancer Lit contains more than 320,000 abstracts of published reports, selected from about 3,000 biomedical and other scientific journals, dealing with all aspects of cancer. Its contents are updated monthly and grow at a rate of more than 40,000 abstracts per year.

Cancer Proj contains more than 21,000 descriptions of current cancer research projects around the world. It also contains more than 4,000 cancer-related projects from mor than 60 different countries outside the USA. Included are descriptions of both federally and privately funded grants and contracts, which are updated every 3 months.

Clin Prot summaries 1,200 clinical cancer therapy protocols supported by the Division of Cancer Treatment of the National Cancer Institute or by cancer centers outside the USA. Any protocol can be retrieved according to the type of cancer, type of agents used, investigator's name, protocol identification numbers, and several other computer-search fields. Through a hook-up with a terminal at the National Library, searches can be entered at any location. Requested information can be viewed at local terminals or printouts mailed from the computer center.

An organization can become a search center by applying to the ICRDB program of the National Library of Medicine for an on-line access code. Required equipment includes a commercially available teletypewriter or a TV-like terminal and teleprinter coupled to a standard telephone line.

The ICRDB program also produces two major types of publications:

(1) *Cancergrams,* which provide researchers with abstracts of recently published results directly related to their current research projects and selected from about 3,000 biomedical journals and other sources. There are more than 60 different cancergrams, each with monthly issues containing 30 to 100 abstracts covering a specific research topic. Researchers in more than 60 nations describe current research projects in a special listing.

(2) *Oncology overviews* contain selected abstracts of published literature. These publications are designed to rapidly update research knowledge of current research topics.

There should be cooperation between different societies and organizations like the Roentgen Society of North America (RSNA), Chronic Leukemia Group B (CLGB), The National Cancer Institute (NCI) and the National Institutes of Health (NIH). Duplication of sources is a waste of time and money and must be avoided.

Crusade against Quacks

Quackery in medicine is as old as the art of healing. Cancer in particular has a tremendous emotional impact and is fertile soil for quackery because of the lack of solid facts and overwhelming fear during prolonged and complicated management. Cancer patients are easy prey to quacks because they always offer more promising simplified alternatives. The medical profession has a long list of visible and invisible opponents; complicating matters is the picture patients have of physicians as intentionally misinforming and ultimately misguiding them. Physicians have even been accused of conspiring against the welfare of sick people. False stories are propagated with testimonials given to support them. Unfortunately, unqualified remarks by the media or immature reports by any authority, or even the scientific media may indirectly help to promote unorthodox modalities of management. Unscrupulous physicians also help to increase mistrust in the medical profession. The inadequacy of some present modalities is sometimes presented to medically uninformed and uneducated public as proof of the shaky situation of the medical profession relative to cancer.

What makes the situation even worse is the physician's self-righteousness; their rigid attitude helps quacks reach their objectives. All this happens at a time when there is no available information or facts to disprove these false endeavors. Innocent, defenseless victims are always attracted to what is pictured as the least complicated procedure, without really having the capability to make a proper judgement regarding choice. The road is paved for proponents of unorthodox methods of treatment, as they offer more promising alternatives. Moreover, they present witnesses to what they claim, in a very personalized approach, which is very hard to beat. They also manage to further alienate patients from their physicians, most of the time by shaking their confidence and encouraging them to defy the medical profession. They always raise false slogans: 'Be your own doctor' and 'Freedom of choice'. Patients remain unaware of either their meaning or impact.

Action against quackery is required in the form of legislation or by informing the public about this threat before valuable time, money, and lives are lost. Personalized contact at all times, if given to the patient with respect to his feelings, probably could avert this trend. Information should be spread on behalf of and under the guidance of the medical profession. What makes the fight against quackery more difficult is that modern quacks are different from the old-time quacks, who used to travel in colorful wagons, dressed differently, and spoke a peculiar language with characteristic style. People did not take them seriously and their audience was small, so that their ambition and scope were limited. Today the situation is entirely different. Quacks use scientific language, are able to capture their audience, and it is very difficult to cite them as pushers of unorthodox modalities. Most of the time, the quacks are not strangers to the scientific milieu. They do not sell oil extracts from different animals as in the past, but do sell compounds with sophisticated formulas. They are outspoken and able to convince their educated audiences. What makes the problem even worse is that they mix business with science, presenting new modalities that cater to people's needs with their strong reasoning for the usefulness of these modalities. This combination of business and science is hard to resist; no doubt, quackery is a very lucrative business that takes advantage of people's suspicions and fears, shining a gleam of hope during these dark times of life. Quacks lack moral fiber; they have only the hope of financial benefit and an irresistible greed for money. They are always organized and influential, rich and hard to oppose. Sometimes they look harmless and are hard to locate or fight.

Quackery is medical fraud, and although it is sometimes harmless, it does keep patients from seeking medical advice in the early stages of their disease. As a result, valuable time is lost – time that could be very precious for the successful management of a potentially curable cancer. Neither the toxicity of the drug nor the harm done, as there may not be any, are as important as the loss of large amounts of money without any real benefit. A positive attitude should be created and propagated among people to enlighten them. Active participation in one's own health care helps prevent alienating the patient. Banning the sale of materials not proven to be scientifically and professionally effective should be enforced by different authorities to protect helpless victims. The crusade against quacks should continue, as they always come back through any weakness in any line of management, with different slogans or different attitudes or ideas.

An important issue is that we should not be confused in differentiating between fighting quackery and promoting new ideas. In considering new ideas as unorthodox treatment methods, we may unknowingly be blocking a new and important breakthrough. History is full of important advances which, at the time of the inception, were considered as unorthodox and unacceptable and consequently were strongly opposed. Every new idea should be scrutinized and studied carefully before it receives publicity or is discredited. Megavitamins, total metabolic therapy, enzyme tablets, nutritional therapy, chelated minerals, and hyperthermal machines are examples of different modalities with no obvious specific effect in the present management of cancer and may be taken, by different people, to be beneficial in the definitive management of cancer, as announced by Dr. *Stephen Barret* of the Lehigh Valley Committee against Health Fraud.

The Role of Different Organizations

Different voluntary organizations can play an important role in propagating the correct information and knowledge among the public; in addition, they can provide different kinds of required services.

The American Cancer Society, first organized by physicians in 1913 to serve patients, their families, the public, and professionals, is the largest voluntary organization. In 1930, it started as the American Society for the Control of Cancer, a time when the American College of Surgeons was asked to help develop standards to provide services for the diagnosis and treatment of cancer. In 1945, lay persons joined physicians in the same corporation with an increase in the financial support. This was also a landmark that indicated that medical problems, because of the accompanying socio-economic implications, are a concern of society as a whole, not only the medical profession. Further expansion followed so that at the present time, there are 58 divisions providing various services. Of $ 118 million collected from voluntary contributors, $ 30 million are used for research grants and residency programs promoting medical schools and undergraduate teaching levels. The American Cancer Society also promotes and upgrades professional cancer education in medical schools. Grants are also given to visiting nurse associations to promote home visits to needy patients. Homemakers and home health aids are also provided. Transportation of patients undergoing radiation treatments, chemotherapy, or rehabilitation, and health aids are provided. Rehabilitation programs such as esophageal speech for laryngectomized patients, cancer clubs in different sectors of society, factories, schools, churches, reaching large aggregations of people needing cancer education are also provided, along with pamphlets, 16-mm movies, posters, exhibits, brochures, magazines, commercials on radio and television, as well as newspaper ads.

The society promotes different screening programs in coordination with community hospitals.

In 1951, the famous campaign against cigarette smoking was launched by the society. They investigated the relationship between smoking and lung cancer and finally came out with the Horn-Hammond report which announced the close relationship between the two. After that came the long and bitter controversy with cigarette companies. In 1964, the Surgeon General's report on smoking and health was published, requesting physicians and dentists to adopt an exemplary role to stop cigarette smoking.

Different institutions also help in cancer education. The NCI is sponsoring an education and training program for surgical oncology. Other societies such as the American College of Radiology and others like the American Society of Therapeutic Radiologists and Roentgenologic Society of North America are sponsoring different programs to promote radiation therapy, setting guidelines for quality control.

References

1   Benedict, W.F., et al.: Inhibition of chemically induced morphological transformation and reversion of the transformed phenotype of ascorbic acid in C_3H 110T½ cells. Cancer Res. *1:* 2796–2801 (1980).

2   Weinstein, B.: The scientific basis for carcinogen detection and primary cancer prevention. Cancer, N.Y. *47:* 1133–1144 (1981).

Detection of Asymptomatic Cases: Screening for Cancer

Organized efforts to detect early cancer were started in the late 1940s under the auspices of the American Cancer Society. In the early 1950s, a committee for cancer detection was formed when preliminary screening programs were followed by improvements in survival rates of patients with cancer of the breast. The 10-year survival rate rose from 44% before 1950 to above 50% in the 1950s.

The rationale for cancer screening is to (a) predict when cancer can occur and detect it at an early stage, and (b) prevent other cancer cases from developing. To start a cancer screening program, physicians have to report their suspicions of a certain trend in the incidence of cancer in a certain location. The patient's history is as good as the physical examination in spotting a cancer-cause relationship. On two occasions, history taking proved to be the only reason for probing and screening for the relationship between cancer and certain predisposing factors. For example, the use of stilbestrol and its relationship to endometrial carcinoma and the relationship of genital infection to herpes and its association with cancer of the cervix were discovered mainly by history taking. An etiologic hypothesis postulates the reason for the suspected increase in cancer incidence. Epidemiologists have to design and plan screening programs to identify individuals at highest risk and to confirm the hypothesis, while, at the same time find a solution to the problem. Intensive education is necessary for the group to be screened to prepare them for these programs and is mandatory for their success. Education may also be extended even to those who are not to be screened, and continued between screening sessions.

To make the screening programs more effective it may be advisable to broaden the definition of high-risk individuals. The potentiating effect of different carcinogens should be taken into account when high-risk individuals are to be defined. This would include race, family history, occupation, geographic location, presence of precancerous conditions and different personal habits. The yield of cancer detection may be low and the cost of screening high, but in the long run, cancer prevention will be more successful.

Conditions Necessary for the Success of Screening Programs

It is impractical to screen the entire population, so good sampling is necessary. The groups to be screened must be properly chosen on the basis of age, sex and, probably, race. Workers in certain occupations and people with certain habits have to be considered.

To evaluate the effectiveness of screening programs and to detect cancer in its asymptomatic phase, the people screened must be asymptomatic. To justify screening programs, the detection rate should be high. One successful way to ensure a good turn-out is to send out letters, preferably for, and signed by the family physician. Because of the usual good rapport between patient and physician this was found to insure the highest response rate. It was found that 82% of people responded to physician's letters, a greater response than if the letters had been sent out by a person unknown to them. Self-referred persons should be excluded, as most of them have symptoms that could influence the results of the screening program.

Screening programs should be simple and easy to apply on a large scale. Examination room surroundings and screening places should be pleasant, with the privacy of the person ensured. Reporting the test results immediately is appreciated by the persons screened. It should be understood that at screening time cycles of tension and relief run parallel to the screening cycles. Results must be reliable and confidential. Positive results should be dealt with carefully, and further management should be promptly planned. False-positive results would create unnecessary anxiety; therefore, it is necessary to confirm the diagnosis by repeating the test to avoid unwarranted reactions.

Cost-Effectiveness

To generalize cancer screening programs for the entire population is very costly because the cancer detection rate would be 1 per 1,000. Screening programs should be inexpensive and executed by well-trained paramedicals along with volunteers to reduce the cost without compromising results. Volunteers should constitute the majority of the team; professionals should be consulted only as required. Funding by different contributors with supervision and assistance provided by different organizations such as the American Cancer Society would be a great help in reducing the total cost. Using community hospitals and similar places helps to reduce spending. Doing more than one test during a single visit increases productivity. Needless to say, the choice of high-risk groups is the most important factor in improving cost-effectiveness. One drawback of the screening program is that persons with negative results may discount subsequent signs or symptoms as non-cancerous and people should be strongly warned against this. The value of any screening program has to be assessed in terms of prolonged survival, decreased mortality, and optimal cost-effectiveness. The results should be evaluated as a whole, with all relevant factors considered, as for example, a change in mortality for cancer of the cervix is related not only to screening programs and Pap smears, but to changes in the effect of risk factors, socio-economic differences, sexual practices, and new treatment methods. We must realize that prolonged survival through screening is complicated by the problem of lead time – the time between the detection in the asymptomatic phase and the onset of symptoms – which is equal to the asymptomatic phase. If the patient's life is prolonged only for a time equal to the lead time, then there is no real advantage to a screening program. Some people feel that money should be spent on other trial programs to improve the survival rate and quality of life, which would be more beneficial than the results obtained from screening programs. The greatest benefit of a screening program would be best seen in a fast-growing tumor, where every day counts because the tumor is expected to spread further and survival would be adversely affected by the late detection. The high-risk person who is known to respond as a participant in a screening program is usually an older, wealthier person with more dependents; a high detection rate is expected in this group. The difficulty of getting all high-risk patients into a screening campaign suggests that screening be included and considered a necessary part of routine medical care. Physicians would probably have to be oriented to the program. Low-income classes, where a high detection rate is suspected, do not seem to respond well to these programs, mainly because of their lack of education, helplessness, or lack of continued medical care. Generally speaking, the success or failure of a screening program has an emotional impact on the public just as some cancers do. Accordingly, some people may respond to certain screening programs more enthusiastically than to others. It is unnecessary to screen for cancer that has a low incidence of occurrence, a low detection rate and does not affect the incidence of cancer deaths. Detection of cancer can be achieved by two methods:

(1) Annual physical and dental examination. In a study by cancer detection centers at the University of Minnesota, over the 21-year period 1948–1969, 23 persons who have had repeat physical examinations were

found to have asymptomatic cancer. Although this is a very low detection rate, it can be improved by increased public awareness and scrupulous medical examinations.

(2) Periodic screening programs should be emphasized for the common forms of cancer, screening for the earliest visible or detectable changes. Screening for specific tumor markers and biochemical changes are not fully developed methods but may be useful in the future. Screening programs for immunologic defects and chromosomal aberrations need to be improved further. A few of the screening programs will be discussed in detail as they represent special interesting problems for large segments of the population.

Screening for Cancer of the Breast

There are four screening tests that can be used for the early detection of cancer of the breast: (a) breast self-examination (BSE); (b) physical examination; (c) mammography; (d) thermography.

The need for early diagnosis in cancer of the breast is obvious from various studies; 80% of breast cancers detected in screening programs had no regional lymph node involvement. Of those who were found to have lymph node involvement, 89% survived 5 years. The overall survival rate of cases detected by screening programs was 95.6%, and the 10-year survival was 81%, substantially better than what is generally reported for the survival of patients with cancer of the breast.

Breast Self-Examination

Little is known about the efficiency of BSE in the diagnosis of breast cancer. A survey from Canada indicated that only 36% of Canadian women were examining themselves regularly each month. In a limited trial where benefits and methods of doing the BSE were explained, 90% were able to perform the examination competently and with confidence. The NCI is supporting a program to help women throughout the country learn to do the BSE. As most women see breast cancer as a major health threat, BSE may become a useful modality for early detection. Some women may feel nervous and are obviously afraid of performing the BSE, because they fear missing a lump, or they are afraid to palpate a lump in their own breasts. About 20% of women have no confidence in their ability to do a BSE and are nervous about practicing it. In women who never did BSE, it was found that their tumor, when it was detected, was 5 cm or larger. Yet among those who regularly practiced BSE and found tumors, these were discovered before they reached 2 cm in size. The present recommendation is that BSE should be done once a month in women over 20 years of age.

Physical Examination

This is usually done annually and is considered by *Leo J. Mahoney* [17] as one of the best available screening tests for the early detection of breast cancer. In view of the current argument about mammography and its suspect risks, screening for breast cancer in women under 35 years of age by physical examination is best, particularly after the Bailey report. *Bailey* contended that mass screening by mammography may benefit only a minority of cases. Statistical models showed that breast cancer detection is only advanced by an average of about 1 year by mammographic screening [5]. Unfortunately, the period during which breast cancer is radiologically detectable but clinically unpalpable is likely to be a relatively short one in the overall natural history of the disease. Mass screening, therefore, may benefit only a minority of cases if mammography alone is done. *Mahoney* contended that, even for high-risk patients, changes in mammograms seem to develop very slowly and recommendations for annual mammographic screening appear to be unwarranted. He also pointed out that of 24 malignant solid lesions first detected clinically, only 4 showed changes on serial mammograms. For the early diagnosis of breast cancer, the more rewarding screening method is the annual breast clinical examination and less frequently mammographies for women whose breasts remain clinically normal. He recommended that breast examination be done separately from mammography since negative mammograms may influence the results of physical examination. If the examinations are to be used in combination, they should be done separately and independently. The examiner should not be influenced or biased by the results of either test, but should conduct each separately and independently of the results of either.

Screening by Mammography

In the HIP (Health Insurance Plan) screening program of the Greater New York area, clinical examination was done at the same time as with mammography. No benefit was detected in screening women of 40–49 years of age as the mortality rate was not affected under the age of 50. Subsequent to the HIP study, the NCI and the American Cancer Society have set up 27 demonstration projects in an endeavor to find justification for recommending cancer breast screening programs for the entire population. Screening was suggested only for selected groups, as epidemiologists in 1975 juxtaposed a lack of evidence of benefit for screening by mammography for women under the age of 50 years.

Mammography has been evaluated for its potential carcinogenic effect, particularly after the National Research Council Advisory on Biological Effects of Ionizing Radiation (BEIR) Committee report in 1972. Extrapolating the results of the BEIR report, epidemiologists concluded that even 1 rad might increase the risk of breast cancer to 7 cases per 1,000 population. The National Academy of Science in England has estimated that for a breast dose of 1 rad, 6 new cases of breast cancer per million population per year would appear in 10 years. In England, it is believed unlikely that any significant risks are involved in mammography using skin doses of less than 1 rad in women under the age of 50 years. Survivors of Hiroshima and Nagasaki – groups of young women irradiated for postpartum mastitis, and young TB patients who were screened repeatedly – all were exposed to appreciable amounts of radiation. The carcinogenic effect was noted predominantly in those who were exposed early in life, usually under the age of 35 years, because the longer span of life allows time for the carcinogenic mutation to develop. Moreover, in the younger age group, because of the increased density of breast tissue, low-dose mammography is less effective in revealing details according to *John Bailar III* [3]. Although in the United States, England, and elsewhere, mammography with a skin dose of less than 1 rad in women over 50 years of age is thought to be unlikely to carry significant risks, the general consensus for women under age 35 is that mass screening by mammography is not warranted. In 1976, the NCI established new restrictions on mammography and recommended that it should not be done before the age of 50 years. In younger patients, routine mammography should be done only in the presence of definite indications. The age of women screened in the Dutch survey was above 50 years, reaching to 64. In the Swedish survey it was done for women above 40 years of age.

Although some feel that the mere linear extrapolation of the effect of high-dose radiation relative to carcinogenicity is not scientifically acceptable, publicity about the adverse effect of radiation had an obvious effect on mammography's acceptance by the public and several physicians. Some other radiologic diagnostic procedures have been similarly affected. *Sam Shapiro* [22], in studying the evidence for screening for breast cancer, pointed out that physicians and women are looking for evidence that screening asymptomatic women, correlates with a decreased mortality rate and not just an increased detection rate of early cancers. However, many physicians are still reluctant to accept the presumptive evidence of early diagnosis as a benefit because of the problem of lead time. Moreover, they suspect that patient selectivity may be a factor in the higher survival rate. The value of periodic breast screening has been tempered until further evidence and benefits are confirmed.

Recently, the dose received to the skin during mammography has been lowered to 0.3 rad with the use of a molybdenum target and compression techniques. In addition, the efficiency with which smaller lesions are detected has been improved four times. The dose to the skin in the Swedish study was 0.1 rad, using a single oblique projection. The Beahrs Committee for the Breast Cancer Distribution Project recommended screening by mammography for all women 50 years of age and older, and for all high-risk women 35–49 years of age, as 1.1% of all breast cancers were found in women under the age of 30 and 30% occurred in women under the age of 50. In that study 3.2% of all cases were initially suspected and 1.7% were discovered with additional mammography views. Of all screened suspected cases, 60% had proven cancer. The proponents of mammography point out that half the cancers detected in this demonstration project were diagnosed by mammography. They claim that carcinoma can be detected by mammography before it is detected clinically. Since the risk-benefit ratio should also be considered, it was studied by *Strax* [23] and *Bywaters and Knox* [4]. In the HIP study, follow-up examinations were made for 10 years, during which time the mortality rate was not affected for women under the age of 50, but was reduced by 50% in women between 50 und 59 years of age and by 23% in women between 60 and 69 years of age. The detection rate of asymptomatic breast cancer was increased to 2.6 cases per 1,000 for the initial and subsequent examinations. The results of the Swedish and Dutch surveys showed that high pickup rates may reach up to 3 cases per 1,000 population in the Swedish screening and up to 7 cases per 1,000 population in the Dutch survey. Clinical examination, in addition to mammography, was used in the Dutch study, but only mammography in the Swedish study. In the former survey 1 in 110 cancers was diagnosed by clinical examination only, but in 57% of proven cancers, a suspicious mammogram was the only indication. *Jakobsson* [15] in his study, proved that a single-view mammogram is a simple, efficient approach to breast cancer screening and mammography is more sensitive than clinical examination in detecting breast cancer, contrary to the HIP study in which findings suggested that mammography is of no benefit to women under the age of 50 years. In both the Swedish and Dutch groups, 66–87% of cases had no detectable nodal metastasis – compared to a 75% detection rate in the HIP study – and 10.5% were found to be noninvasive. In the HIP study, in more than 15% of detected carcinomas the size of the tumor was less than 1 cm, but other studies indicated that one of six cancers detected were nonpalpable tumors and one-third of the breast cancers detected through screening would have been missed without mammography.

The time between screening mammographies varied according to different programs and with age. The frequency of mammography screening would essentially have to depend on the lead time. In the HIP study, it was found to be 1 year. But the optimal frequency is unknown and it is uncertain whether the same frequency of screening should be applied to all women. The probability that cancer can develop between screenings makes it even more difficult to optimize the time. It is agreed that high-risk groups should be handled differently, particularly with close physical examination. High-risk factors are considered to be early menarche, late menopause, a family history of breast cancer, first pregnancy after 27 years of age, no history of breast feeding, and a history of breast cancer in the opposite breast. Other factors such as obesity and the use of birth control pills are related to age and onset of pregnancy. The cost benefit has to be evaluated further as screening programs for all women are very expensive at the present detection rate. As discussed previously we should make the screening program cost more attractive by combining breast screening programs with cervical cancer screening programs, or others.

The cost of the screening done by Dr. *Anderson* at the University of Lund, Malmö, Sweden, was $ 2,000.00 per detected cancer, much less expensive than the cost per case detected in the HIP study. In Dr. *Anderson's* study [2], the detection rate was considered to be efficacious in finding early cancer with a low incidence of axillary node involvement. Single-view mammography with cytologic confirmation of suspicious cases by fine needle aspiration biopsy (FNAB), without physical examination, was used by *Jakobsson* to decrease the cost of screening an unselected population to $ 2,860.00. He confirmed that for a total cost of $ 5,000.00 women over the age of 40 years would have a 99% chance of 5 years' survival [15]. The added cost of aspiration biopsy is $ 30 to 60. That is in addition to a nonprofit mammography with a modest additional expense which would accrue for a small number of surgical procedures. *Jakobsson* concluded that breast cancer screening of women over 40 years of age, previously thought to be prohibitively expensive in most Western societies, now seems possible in countries with the highest incidence of breast cancer.

The reliability with which biopsy provides better samples of breast tissues after a suspicious mammogram needs to be improved, as 29% of breast biopsies were found to be negative in screening programs. Moreover, the number of needless mastectomies increased.

Thermography

Thermography is a noninvasive procedure with great potential and appeal and could be ideal for screening programs. It is still, to a great extent, nonspecific, with a high prevalence of false-positive and false-negative results. Findings are usually difficult to interpret and because they are not considered reliable as yet, unnecessary numbers of biopsies may result. Recently, a baseline study with thermography demonstrated a definite thermographic pattern for each breast. These patterns were found to be useful for further follow-up studies in which any change must be investigated thoroughly. Thermography could be of great help in screening women under the age of 50 for cancer of the breast. Improved techniques with computerization and improved sensors may revolutionize its use.

Screening for Cancer of the Cervix

Cancer of the cervix is a sex-related disease closely associated with promiscuity, as demonstrated by *Martin Field* [6]. Although sexual promiscuity has been known throughout history, at no time has it reached such a degree of unrestrained relationships between young people. This change has been described as the sexual revolution, with physical, emotional, and sexual impacts. It is obvious when facing this phenomenon that sex education is deficient and unable to cope with the situation. At present, sex education involves only the teaching of contraception and abortion, with no mention of promiscuity and its complications in relationship to cancer.

The problem of adolescent sexuality and paramarriage are becoming of increasing concern as the mean age of patients with cancer of the cervix in a sexually promiscuous society is becoming lower than in more conservative societies. The other risk factors related to the development of cancer of the cervix include the number of pregnancies and age at first intercourse.

Screening the entire population is expensive and impractical; some even look at it as unjustified. Advocates of cervical screening see it as a fundamental method in preventing cancer of the cervix; others doubt its benefit and wonder if money could be spent on more productive areas of patient care. Yet screening for cancer of the cervix is different from screening for cancer of the breast. First and most important, no hazard is involved. The second reason is that squamous cell carcinoma of the cervix is a final stage of increasing dysplasia of the cells which may be caused by a virus or disease transmitted during promiscuous sexual activity. It is possible to demonstrate these various stages and prevent their progress before they reach the infiltrative stage, at which point they penetrate beyond the basement membrane of the cell.

The precancerous changes can be detected and stopped. Moreover, it is easier to detect early cancerous stages, which are more curable. Screening for cancer of the cervix by the Papanicolaou smear has been extensively used in the USA since the 1940s, and available data generally support its value. Cytologic examination can also detect cancer of the lung, urinary bladder, stomach, colon, and oral cavity. But, it is most successful in detecting cancer of the cervix because of the ease with which the procedure can be performed routinely during physical examination. No additional work, hospitalization, anesthesia, or minor surgical procedure is needed, it has no complications, and it can be done routinely on a large scale.

It is clear that screening the cervix is an ideal demonstration of the effectiveness and use of a screening program. Again, questions arise as to whether a screening program increases the tumor detection rate or decreases the death rate. Several screening programs have documented, statistically, a significant fall in the incidence of cervical cancer and its death rate. But, the impact of different screening programs on the mortality rate varies from country to country because of several factors. In England and Wales, the mortality rate was already falling before screening programs were adopted. The reduction was due to improved treatment techniques and a better understanding of the behavior of cancer of the cervix. The application of more appropriate treatment methods, other than surgery, became available with the development of modern radiotherapy.

It was difficult to demonstrate an additional drop in the mortality rate until 10 years after the application of screening programs. Obviously, there is a hidden advantage in applying screening programs despite the equal death rate, as survivors of cancers detected in screening programs showed no morbidity after the precancerous condition was treated. Every patient treated for invasive cancer will become sterile, whether treated by surgery or radiotherapy. Without a doubt, it is better to prevent cancer of the cervix than to apply more efficient treatment modalities as they still carry a certain morbidity.

In other countries, where management has not been proven, the mortality rate showed a remarkable drop with the introduction of the Pap smear screening program. In British Columbia, all sexually active women over 20 years of age were screened and the incidence rate, was demonstrated by 17 years of screening, was reduced by 33%. In Toledo, Ohio, a 66% reduction in the incidence rate was obvious when 90% of those at risk were screened. In Louisville, Ky., 94% of the population at risk has been screened since 1967, and from 1955 to 1978 a 57% decrease in incidence and a 51% drop in mortality rate has been observed. In Auckland, New Zealand, when only 20% of the women at risk were screened, the mortality rate, which was already falling before the start of the screening campaign, did not show an accelerated response. One benefit of screening programs in dealing with cancer of the cervix is the increase in the number of in situ lesions detected and the obvious reversal in the ratio of early to advanced disease. In the United Kingdom, although the total number of deaths is small, the death rate from cervical cancer in women below the age of 35 years is rising.

The cost of screening millions of women, when compared with the benefit of saving a small proportion of lives, is a controversial topic. Despite the ease with which the Pap smear can be performed, the cost of generalizing these programs is prohibitive, the yield is relatively low, and the drop in mortality rate is not that noticeable. Screening the entire population may be a factor in diluting the detection rate, and gives the impression that the effect of these programs is not that significant. Therefore, these programs must be limited to high-risk groups where the yield of detected cancer will obviously be higher than that in the general population. The issue is to identify this high-risk group by using certain criteria as the incidence of cancer of the cervix is higher among (1) low socioeconomic classes; (2) early age of sexual activity; (3) promiscuity.

History of Genital Herpes Infection

The correlation between cervical carcinoma and the herpes type II virus was suspected after the incidence of premalignant cervical lesions was found to be high in women who had the virus infection before, and reached a 23% involvement rate as 39 of 166 persons examined showed these changes.

Data from the Massachusetts Department of Public Health showed that the effectiveness of cervical screening programs cannot be substantiated when age, rather than categorization of high-risk groups is considered [18]. That issue was discussed to demonstrate screening problems in general, as the question of screening the wrong women was raised. If most of the screening was done in young persons who are at much less risk, it would reflect poorly on the efficiency and productivity of screening programs. The recommendation of the British Society of Cytologists is that screening women below the age of 30 years should be selective. Abnormal cytology, studied by Dr. *Martin Fieldman* [7], was found in 70.8 Pap smears per 1,000 teenagers screened. Examination by experienced colposcopists helps to recognize false-positives and carcinoma in situ. The probability that an invasive lesion will be discovered in a teenager is so remote that some investigators question the need for routine cytologic screening in this age group. The detection of intraepithelial disease is very important as the progress of change can be controlled, the occurrence of invasive carcinoma can be prevented, and more aggressive management for invasive cancer of the cervix, which could cause sterility, can be avoided. When intraepithelial changes are diagnosed, the patient is seen after 3 months, but after three consecutive normal Pap smears, the intervals are lengthened and the patient is then seen after 6 months and subsequently longer intervals thereafter. It is unjustified to follow patients with mild or moderate dysplasia, unless it persists or progresses.

The Chicago Board of Health has reduced the number of Pap smears taken in women under the age of 19 years, unless they are epidemiologically and/or clinically warranted. The incidence of invasive cancer in teenagers is generally rare; only 25 cases were reported in the literature since 1862, according to *C. Fields* [8]. Another study by *G. H. Friedell* [9] commented on the need for routine Pap smears. After examining smears from teenage girls, he mentioned that perhaps the best solution would be to consider the biologic age of the cervix rather than the teenager's chronologic age. He developed an equation in which the biologic age of the cervix equals the girl's age $+ K_f$ (K_f is the number of years of active sex life before the age of 20). Therefore, when $K_f = 5$ or more, a smear must be taken and when K_f is less than 5, a smear need not be taken. With this formula, it seems likely that cervical smears would only be required for a relatively small number of teenagers.

In a 7-year retrospective analysis from Chicago, the Board of Health Cancer Control Section screened 33,641 teenagers. 58% or 1.7 per 1,000 had abnormal cytology, Class III, IV, or V. In Chicago, screening from 1962 through 1969 showed that approximately 25% of screened persons were teenagers, with an extremely low yield of suspected Class III and IV.

The problem of mailing smear tests is sometimes controversial, as results seem to disagree with other repeated tests. In addition, patients with negative mailed smears had later developed invasive cervical carcinoma. Clearly, a Pap smear during gynecologic examination is much more reliable.

The issue is to encourage more older women, particularly those at high risk, to attend screening programs, to undergo cervical cytology examination, and to continue doing so in postmenopausal life, as shown by *Donald Ostergord* [19]. Yet postmenopausal women who already had had several negative smears throughout their reproductive years are very unlikely to develop cancer of the cervix at this age. The frequency with which Pap smears are taken varies according to risk factors; hence, an annual test is not recommended for low-risk women, and only the regular gynecologic examination need be done. Intervals between Pap smear examinations should be distant for those at low risk, and a period of 3 years or longer is recommended before the test is repeated. If two successive Pap smears from women over 18 years of age are negative, the interval between these examinations should be gradually prolonged.

To properly evaluate the significance of abnormal cytology, colposcopy is recommended to rule out invasive carcinoma in suspected cases [19]. In advanced dysplasia, colposcopy may decrease the need for cervical biopsies and conization [26]. During pregnancy, abnormal cytology should be evaluated with great care and management varied according to the stage of pregnancy. In high-risk patients the Pap smear should be taken annually, and with any abnormal cytology it should be repeated in 3 months or less.

Classifying sexually active or promiscuous women as high-risk creates problems because it is met with abject refusal and objections. They fear a loss of confidentiality, which makes them resist attending screening programs. The remedy is to assure their privacy and provide discrete examining rooms.

Screening for Cancer of the Colon

Cancer of the colon is the second leading cause of death from cancer, exceeded only by the mortality rate for cancer of the lung. Death from cancer of the colon accounts for 15% of all cancer deaths.

In the United States 100,000 cases of colorectal cancer were detected in 1976; 70,000 cancers of the colon and 30,000 rectal cancers. At present, the mortality rate from cancer of the colon is increasing relative to the mortality rate for rectal cancer [11]. Over half of people with colorectal carcinoma are expected to die, mainly because their disease was discovered late. Different studies showed that 90% of early lesions of colorectal cancer can be cured with proper management. As survival rates remained the same for several decades, it became obvious that the early discovery of colorectal disease is the key to the problem. 90% of intestinal cancer occurs at the age of 52 years or older; individuals under the age of 40 who develop colorectal cancer are more likely to have a family history of colonic cancer. Unfortunately, no chromosomal anomaly can be cited and used as a diagnostic or prognostic marker, such as the Philadelphia chromosome, which is used as an indicator in chronic granulocytic leukemia. Cancer-complicating hereditary disease is described in different syndromes such as Gardner's syndrome, Peutz-Jeghers syndrome, familial adenomatosis, or complicating inflammatory bowel disease. In familial adenomatosis of the colon and rectum, the progressive phase of abnormal growth changes can be observed and may be present in different areas at the same time, accompanied by a change in the enzyme composition in the cells of the colon.

Cancer of the colon can be detected early if high-risk persons are identified and examined periodically for tissue enzymes. Proper management should be provided with the earliest changes. The behavior of this disease in its early stage is predictable and management can be tailored according to expectations. In other cases, the association between malignancies of the bowel and those of the skin is known. Physicians should be familiar with the skin changes that signal the presence of an internal malignancy. Cancer of the colon in older patients is not suspected to be familial or hereditary. Theories about diet-related causes have been suggested. The incidence of colonic cancer was also noticed to vary according to geographic areas and socioeconomic factors. As the disease is more prevalent in some countries and in certain classes, high-risk patients must be identified before they develop symptoms of the disease.

Once cancer of the colon becomes symptomatic, the survival rate drops to 40% compared to 88% if the disease is diagnosed during its asymptomatic or even at its early symptomatic phase. Unfortunately, symptoms of early colonic cancer are not specific. Such signs as a change in bowel movement habits, abdominal pain, backache, weakness, general tiredness, anemia, loss of appetite, loss of weight, can be easily missed. Physicians alone are not to be blamed for the late discovery of colonic cancer, as the public also may ignore most of these signs and symptoms and discharge them as minor ailments that can be treated symptomatically. Visible blood in stools is a late sign; tests for occult blood will be discussed later. The impact on survival of detecting symptomatic cancer early has been disputed – particularly proponents of mass screening for cancer of the colon, who claim only diagnosis of presymptomatic cancer holds the key to improved survival, claim that early detection would not change the prognosis. Opponents of mass screening for colorectal cancer claim that the benefits of mass screening are not completely appreciated and that the detection rate is not high – only 1% – a result that hinders the enthusiasm to proceed. Their belief is that the diagnosis of early symptomatic colonic cancer gives a better chance for survival if it is treated aggressively, a situation similar to the early diagnosis and treatment of breast cancer. They contend that a delay in diagnosing the symptoms is the main reason for the poor results. Moreover, they believe it is futile to look for asymptomatic colonic cancer, because with combined management, results in early symptomatic cancer of the colon can be much improved. They believe further that money should be spent to improve the results of treatment rather than wasted in detecting presymptomatic cancer.

But the detection and management of existing precancerous conditions – polyps and other benign lesions, which were present in 1–2% of individuals – would be considered a good prophylactic measure. The Minnesota experience has demonstrated that 80–90% of the cancers that could occur in such patients can be avoided. Even those who do develop cancer are potentially curable if followed closely and promptly managed.

Identification of high-risk patients is essential to make the best use of mass screening for cancer of the colon. Comprehensive mass screening of persons over 40 years of age could be maintained at a low profile, depending on clinical judgement. The hemoccult test, which detects hidden blood in the stool, may be very useful in detecting asymptomatic cancer of the colon. The test is inexpensive, simple, aesthetically acceptable and merits further study. *Greegor* [13] advocated a meat-free, high-bulk diet without excess vitamin C for 4 days with the immediate examination of slides for 3 consecutive days. The test is positive in 5% of cases, but only 1% of these cases was found to have asymptomatic cancer. A negative test does not rule out cancer of the colon, but false-negatives are low and can occur with ascorbic acid intake and with bland diets. False-positives are present especially in people on a meat diet and could reach up to 1%. After the hemoccult test was introduced, fewer patients were referred for barium enemas. However, it is not considered a substitute for proctosigmoidoscopy. Unfortunately, the hemoccult test is negative in 83.3% of polyps.

If the hemoccult test is positive, patients are referred for sigmoidoscopic examination and barium enema with air contrast, particularly if the patient is 65 years old or older. If these studies are negative, then a repeat hemoccult test is done in 2 months. If it persists as positive, then colonoscopy should be done. Younger patients with a positive hemoccult should have the test repeated in 2 months before further procedures are done. In asymptomatic patients, $ 500.00 of workup ending in a normal finding in a high percentage of patients is of concern to many. In asymptomatic persons over 50 years of age, the use of fecal occult blood tests, repeated annually, is recommended.

Digital examination in a physical checkup is an expedient way to detect malignancy and is helpful in both cancer of the rectum and prostate. It can detect 12% of large bowel cancers, which, if discovered before it becomes symptomatic, would show a much higher cure rate. Rectal digital examination is recommended as an annual routine procedure in persons over 40 years of age.

Cytologic Examination

Exfoliative cytology assists the diagnosis of esophageal and gastric cancers, pulmonary and genitourinary tumors. However, exfoliative cytology fails to detect an intramural tumor if it is covered by a layer of fibrin [25, 26].

Direct visualization and brush smears with cytologic lavage are also possible, particularly in patients with diffuse premalignant lesions. Cytologic examination of the lower gastrointestinal tract is time-consuming and necessitates good preparation, using cleansing enemas with purgatives. This examination is considered much more complicated than cytologic examination of the stomach and esophagus, where irrigation and lavage yield large clusters of cells for smears prepared from brush specimens. The value of cytologic examination depends largely on its accuracy and specificity. Improved techniques are needed if early diagnosis is to be achieved and priority given to screening highly suspicious, high-risk patients.

Sigmoidoscopy

As 55–70% of colonic cancers occur within the 25-cm sigmoidoscopic range, the entire colon is technically available for examination. In asymptomatic individuals over 40 years of age, cancer can be detected early. Detected by sigmoidoscopy, cancer of the colon has a cure rate of 90% in the 15-year follow-up. Screening by sigmoidoscopy has different problems: its usefulness is limited and it can be done only by experts. Although sigmoidoscopy is the most important single examination in the discovery of polyps and early colorectal cancer, the procedure is not adaptable to mass screening. It is costly in terms of time, manpower, and cost-effect, and people are reluctant to undergo the examination [1].

If physicians would increase their use of sigmoidoscopic examinations, colorectal cancer would be detected earlier. Efforts surely need to be made to encourage people to accept sigmoidoscopic examinations. Of 90% of women scheduled for breast and gynecologic examination, only 42% of the women examined had routine sigmoidoscopy while 54% of physical examinations in men included sigmoidoscopy. Most were done to assess rectal and abdominal complaints and to follow patients after polyp or surgical resection of carcinoma. Even in families with a history of colorectal cancer, 50% had not had a sigmoidoscopic examination. Most of the sigmoidoscopies were performed as a routine procedure; in only 23% were they done as part of a general physical examination. The preparation required, the aesthetic factor, and fear of the procedure, which is uncomfortable or painful, are some of the reasons why people are reluctant to submit to sigmoidoscopy. Patients in high socioeconomic levels often undergo sigmoidoscopy on a regular basis, more often than those in lower socioeconomic classes. The population at large is less aware of it as a screening procedure, unlike screening programs for breast cancer and Pap smears for cervical malignancy.

The obstacles to routine sigmoidoscopy are summarized below and are not attributed to patients alone. *Grant* [12], in his survey, revealed that while 67% of physicians performed sigmoidoscopy, only 14% did so routinely in asymptomatic patients. In another survey, 50% of physicians did not do routine sigmoidoscopy. Many physicians are reluctant to perform sigmoidoscopy as it is time-consuming and costly; sometimes they even lack the necessary equipment. (Surprisingly, 40% of the physicians themselves never underwent sigmoidoscopy.) Others feel that the yield is too small and should be done only if the hemoccult test is positive, although it was found by *Gilberstein* [11] that the detection rate of cancer by proctosigmoidoscopy, in men, was greater than that for cervical smears in women. It was found to be 0.3%, but if patients were symptomatic, the discovery rate was 10 times greater, reaching up to 3%. With minimal training, most physicians should be able to perform it. The procedure can be done in a few minutes, in a variety of positions, is not costly or troublesome and requires minimal specialization. For those who resist the examination, an empathetic explanation and reassurance are helpful.

Incentives should be offered by insurance companies to entice people to have these tests. Education and an explanation about this procedure may encourage more people to have it performed. A very good attitude for the insurance companies would be to ask physicians to fulfill certain requirements for reimbursement. For example, in colonoscopy, the physician's report should include the greatest distance the instrument was introduced and whether the cecum was visualized or not. The description of gross pathologic findings should also be included in the report. An incomplete report should be treated differently. Rigid sigmoidoscopy can be introduced only to 25 cm, but flexible sigmoidoscopy goes up to 40 or 50 cm from the anal verge and can reach 56.4 cm [16], offering a distinct advantage in detecting lesions proximal to the 25-cm limit. Polyps and cancers are more common in the left colon. When sigmoidoscopy was done properly, no adenocarcinoma was reported or pathology did not develop in the interim between repeated annual examinations, particularly in the rectal area. After two initial negative examinations, sigmoidoscopy would be recommended every 3–5 years for persons over 50 years of age.

Fiberoptic Colonoscopy

This is most efficient to detect early, potentially curable cancer of the colon. Half the cancers detected by this procedure were not seen in barium studies. *Gilberstein* [10] reports that colonoscopy is far superior to barium enema for assessing gastrointestinal bleeding and has revolutionized the approach to the diagnosis and management of patients with colorectal neoplasms. It has also simplified the removal of polyps without laparotomy. Brush cytology has been improved so that its yield and the percentage of tissue diagnoses has improved, according to studies by *Sidney J. Winawer et al.* [26]. Barium enema and colonoscopy are of particular help in right-sided colonic cancer. Double-contrast barium enema examination is usually recommended, and full colonoscopy is used for doubtful cases.

Barium Enema

Barium enema is too costly and too time-consuming to be considered a routine screening test for the asymptomatic individual. It should be used as an investigational procedure in symptomatic patients or high-risk individuals. Air study with barium contrast enema are useful before fiberoptic colonoscopy; direct brush or lavage cytology, help to clarify suspicious lesions in areas beyond the reach of standard sigmoidoscopy. Unfortunately, exfoliative cytology is a vastly underutilized technique that could help to detect in situ or early cancer of the colon, especially in patients with ulcerative colitis. But to get reliable satisfactory specimens, the patient must be properly prepped to avoid false-positives or -negatives and to obtain an adequate number of well-preserved cells.

Thomas T. Irving [14] discussed the reason that hinders the enthusiasm to proceed with a screening program. He reported that colorectal cancer does not generate the same emotional appeal as breast cancer and leukemia. Screening for carcinoembryonic antigen (CEA) in the blood does not help to detect cancer of the colon early. Routine screening for CEA in early cancer of the colon revealed that levels are not elevated. Moreover, in benign disease, cirrhosis of the liver, pancreatitis, inflammatory bowel disease, and in heavy smokers, CEA levels may be elevated. This test may only be useful to follow up the management of cancer of the colon by continuously monitoring CEA levels to detect early recurrence. Studies of fecal bulk constituents for ungraded cholesterol, bacterial enzymes, and metabolic breakdown products have been reported by *Reddi* [20] for low- and high-risk patients with colonic problems.

Screening for Gastric Cancer

In relatives of patients with gastric cancer or atrophic gastritis, B_{12} studies should be done do detect further changes. Cytology and gastroscopy may be required to monitor high-risk patients closely. Serum gastrin levels are usually elevated in pernicious anemia, but not with atrophic gastritis where the risk of cancer of the stomach may be particularly high in patients with antral gastritis. Fiberoptic gastroscopy helped to detect asymptomatic gastric cancer early for a cure rate that reached 60%. Cytodiagnosis needs skilled and available expertise for successful exploration, as mentioned by *Wenger et al.* [25]. Gastric cancer is a leading cause of death in Japan, and mass screening by cytologic and endoscopic examinations with a mini-camera led to its early discovery; in 98% of the cases a cure was claimed. CEA, unfortunately, is nonspecific and can be elevated in cancer of the stomach, breast, and endometrium, but predominantly in colorectal-cancer. Other diseases such as nephrotic syndrome as well as other malignancies cause elevated CEA. Consequently, its only use is to monitor follow-up treatments in patients with already known malignancies.

Screening for Cancer of the Lung

Cancer of the lung remains the number-1 cancer killer in the USA. In 1980, the death rate from this disease alone reached 100,000 per year, a rate that approximates the death rate of all accidents and accounts for 22% of all cancer deaths. A chest X-ray and sputum cytology are the only currently available screening tests for presymptomatic lung cancer. Unfortunately, symptoms usually occur at a late stage of the disease, but play only a minor role in its early detection. Asymptomatic cancer may be easier to detect in high-risk people who need to be identified, closely watched, and followed. The risk factors in lung cancer are known to be related to occupational, environmental, and socioeconomic habits.

Cigarette smoking is responsible for more than 80% of all lung cancers, as reported in some series. In asbestos workers, coke oven workers, uranium miners, workers in certain metallic smelting and refining plants and in some branches of the chemical industry the incidence of lung cancer is higher than in other segments of the population. The incidence of cancer of the lung in women has been increasing more rapidly than in men because of recent cigarette smoking problems.

In May 1970, the Division of Thoracic Disease at the Mayo Clinic announced its empiric policy concerning screening for lung cancer. Any person aged 45 years or older who smokes one pack of cigarettes or more each day should have a sputum cytology examination as well as a chest X-ray study at least once a year. The Mayo program (MLP) was established to determine whether a chest X-ray examination every 4 months and sputum cytology for 3 consecutive days in high-risk patients can significantly lower the death rate from lung cancer. Previously unsuspected lung cancers were discovered in 86 of 9,313 persons screened for lung cancer. These cases were detected by X-ray studies more often than by sputum cytology. Moreover, they were not all asymptomatic. The results of this study suggested that radiologic examination every 4 months aided by cytologic screening for lung cancer may benefit the high-risk group.

The results of periodic screening of the population for lung cancer in Philadelphia, have been poor in terms of 5-year survival rates. Among men who developed lung cancer, 84% of cases found by periodic screening after a normal chest X-ray on entry to study had one or more symptoms before cancer was detected.

Sputum Cytology

The yield of positive results is higher when the lesion is located centrally than when it is located peripherally. Even fiberoptic bronchoscopy and brushings for cytologic examination show a lower diagnostic yield for peripheral tumors; a yield parallel to the size of the lesion. Multiple-day cytology has an even greater diagnostic accuracy. However, it is economically impractical to screen the entire adult population periodically; moreover, the test's sensitivity, validity, and cost need to be examined further. Sputum cytology may be negative, in the presence of lung cancer, especially for peripheral lesions, but its use may make earlier detection possible. However, whether a higher cure rate will result has not been confirmed.

Unfortunately, false-positive results can occur in patients with pulmonary infarcts and other benign diseases [21]. The annual cost of chest X-ray studies and cytologic examinations of sputum at 6-month intervals would be over $ 70.00 per person. By itself, the cytologic diagnosis of lung cancer may be misleading and should be considered for each patient, individually, helped by other results.

On the whole, sputum cytology for the early detection of lung cancer has not been encouraging, and deaths from this disease appear to be unaffected by X-ray examinations and sputum cytology in asymptomatic high-risk persons. Preventive measures are still being sought to decrease the mortality rate. However, until sufficient controlled data have been accumulated and been critically analyzed, it is not wise to accept the results of scattered early studies. Conclusion must leave some room for more definite future data. At the present time, strenuous efforts should be directed towards preventive measures.

It was predicted that the greatest reduction in mortality rate could be achieved if cigarette smoking ceased, but additional benefits would be obtained by reducing exposure to other environmental and occupational respiratory carcinogens. According to the Surgeon General's 1980 report, more women than men between the ages of 17 and 24 years are smoking, and this report predicts that by 1983 more women will die from lung cancer than from breast cancer. There is hope that a vaccine that would benefit high-risk individuals or the postoperative patient in whom a malignant tumor has been removed can be developed. Different known health hazards should be promptly eliminated. For example, asbestos has been known to be associated with cancer of the lung for at least 40 years. Yet the incidence of diffuse malignant mesothelioma continued to rise because of the marked increase in the use of asbestos in the shipbuilding industry, as insulation in different merchandise and machines, and its use around pipes. The synergistic effect of different carcinogens, due to combined exposure to airborne hazards such as car fumes and cigarette smoke and occupational carcinogens, should be realized and must be continually monitored in workers in different industries and people in different geographic locations. Healthy air standards have to be maintained and people should be continually advised of the quality of the air they breathe.

References

1   Abramson, D.J.: Sigmoidoscopy in women: comparison with breast and gynecologic examinations in 1,000 patients. Ca 28: 202–219 (1978).

2   Anderson, I.: Breast cancer screening with mammography. A population based randomized trial with mammography as the only screening method. Radiology 132: 273–276 (1979).

3   Bailar, J., III: Screening for early breast cancer. Cancer, N.Y. 39: 2783–2795 (1977).

4   Bywaters, J.L.; Knox, E.G.: The organization of breast cancer services. Lancet i: 849–851 (1976).

5   Canadian Medical Association: Mass survey and treatment of carcinoma of the cervix. A retrospect report. Can. med. Ass. J. 116: 1003–1012 (1976).

6   Field, M.: Abnormal cytology in the teenagers. Am. J. Obstet. Gynec. 126: 418–421 (1976).

7   Fieldman, M.: Intraepithelial neoplasia of the uterine cervix in the teenager. Cancer, N.Y. 41: 1405–1408 (1978).

8   Fields, C.: Experience in Pap smear and cytological observation of teenage girls. Am. J. Obstet. Gynec. 124: 731–734 (1976).

9   Friedell, G.H.: Cancer of the cervix, a selective review. Pathol. A. 1: 48 (1966).

10   Gilberstein, V.A.: Colonoscopy in the detection of carcinoma of the intestine. Surgery Gynec. Obstet. 149: 877–878 (1979).

11   Gilberstein, V.A.: Proctosigmoidoscopy and polypectomy in reducing the incidence of rectal cancer. Cancer, N.Y. 34: 936–939 (1974).

12   Grant, R.N.: Continued education in cancer for the physicians in the United States – an appraisal. Acta Un. int. Cancr. *19–67:* 970 (1963).

13   Greegor, D.H.: Occult blood testing for detection of asymptomatic colon cancer. Cancer, N.Y. *28:* 131–134 (1971).

14   Irving, T.T.: Delay in diagnosis of symptomatic colorectal cancer (Letter). Lancet *i:* 489 (1979).

15   Jakobsson, L.B.: Single view mammography, a simple and efficient approach to breast cancer screening. Cancer, N.Y. *38:* 1124–1129 (1976).

16   Lipshutz, G.R., et al.: Flexible sigmoidoscopy as a screening procedure for neoplasm of the colon. Surgery Gynec. Obstet. *148:* 19–22 (1979).

17   Mahoney, L.J.: Annual clinical examination: the best available screening test for breast cancer. New Engl. J. Med. *301:* 315–316 (1979).

18   Massachusetts Department of Health: Papanicolau testing: are we screening the wrong women? New Engl. J. of Med. *294:* 223 (1976).

19   Ostergord, D.: Evaluation of abnormal cervical cytology during pregnancy with colposcopy. Am. J. Obstet Gynec. *134:* 756–758 (1979).

20   Reddi, B.: Metabolic epidemiology of large bowel cancer: fecal bulk and constituents of high risk North American and low risk Finnish population. Cancer, N.Y. *42:* 2832–2838 (1978).

21   Scoggins, W., et al.: False positive cytological diagnosis of lung carcinoma in patients with pulmonary infarcts. Ann. thor. Surg. *24:* 474–480 (1977).

22   Shapiro, S.: Evidence of screening for breast cancer from randomized trial. Cancer, N.Y. *39:* 2772–2782 (1977).

23   Strax, P.: The present status of mammography. Med. Times, N.Y. *95:* 46 (1967).

24   Strax, P., et al.: Mammography and clinical examination in mass screening for cancer of the breast. Cancer, N.Y. *20:* 2184–2188 (1967).

25   Wenger, J., et al.: Cancer clinical aspects. Gastroenterology *61:* 598–605 (1971).

26   Winawer, S.J., et al.: Colonoscopic biopsy and cytology in the diagnosis of colon cancer. Cancer, N.Y. *42:* 2849–2853 (1978).

Chapter 8

Changing Concepts in Cancer Management

Since the dawn of history, the art of healing has evolved along with ancient cultures. It varied from one civilization to another, but most of the time herbal remedies were used. Relative advances showed in some countries more than in others, yet the prevalent idea was that magic and the curse of evil spirits could bring or avert disease through the *magic* man or the priest. Fire, leeches, and extracts from different animals as well as trips to distant places were used as cures. Over the years the art of healing became more complicated. Different drugs were introduced. Healers were known to be cultured people who were sometimes philosophers or astronomers and were looked upon with respect. Gradually, medicine, as practiced by professionals, became more sophisticated, while advances in technology helped its rapid maturation as a science, different specialities were established, and various schools of thoughts laid the foundation for modern medicine. At the present time, physicians are highly educated people, viewed with admiration and respect by society as a whole. They were, until recently, viewed as demigods and their words were taken as gospel without hesitation. The publicity afforded through the medical media, with its diverse lines of management, together with obvious trends advocated by different centers, all added to the lay public's confusion as to what was right and what was wrong. Patients have obviously become hesitant about the choice of management. New legislation was passed to protect the patient's rights to know, to choose, and to decide.

In Massachusetts, a patient's bill of rights was announced by the American Hospital Association (AHA) Board of Trustees, Committee on Health Care, House of Delegates, on February 6, 1973. This bill called for the patient's right to obtain information about his diagnosis, his disease, and the right to refuse any treatment in addition to that provided. Patient privacy and confidentiality were to be assured. The physician-patient relationship, although it basically remained the same, was complicated by obvious changes so that the physician's job also changed. Prescribing or recommending a certain procedure may be met with some reluctance by the patient and patient's family. Thus the physician is now burdened with the responsibility of providing good medicine while, at the same time, being confronted with the added new challenge of selling his skills and promoting his own ideas over those of others to a patient already confused by what is available. Consequently, the patient simply cannot make a clear decision.

A cancer patient is usually overwhelmed by the rapid succession of events. His ability to make a sound judgment is therefore curtailed and may in fact be influenced by the emotional impact of what he or she had read or heard. Moreover, a cancer patient may have read different reports about unnecessary surgery by different physicians. Interviews of women in an NCI study revealed that 63% felt that physicians sometimes removed breasts unnecessarily. Consequently, they become reluctant to accept, without further questioning, what the physician plans to do, and need to be convinced as well as assured that the care being offered is the best available.

This is why it is advisable for a physician to explain the role of different aspects of management in simple rather than technical terms without withholding pertinent information from the patient or, at the same time, providing erroneous facts. The patient's right to seek a second opinion has further complicated the physician-patient relationship. However, *second opinions* are becoming more fashionable and increasingly popular, although 30% of patients do not want to let their physicians know that they have been seeking a second opinion.

The patient's right to choose is a very controversial issue, but one that must be respected, although not to the extent it compromises management. It is incumbent on the physician to make it easy for the patient and his family to make such a choice, by properly informing them of the advantage of different modalities without bias, which is a very difficult task. The hospital-based tumor board is an ideal medium for the discussion of different opinions, and to exchange different information so that an objective, unbiased decision can be reached. A continued dialogue between different specialists should be reflected in management planning. Differences in opinion should not be revealed to the patients, as they could confuse them and thereby have a negative effect. It was found that highly educated younger women with a high income usually seek more choice in their line of management. The presence of other approved methods as recognized lines of management made the choice for lay people more difficult. Even professionals who lean toward the use of their own modality are experiencing some difficulty in admitting to the use of other methods. The promotion of these new modalities was basically to implement and improve surgical results. Their obvious effectiveness in the management of cancer, as a separate modality, was proved over the years; different studies attested to their effectiveness so that their acceptance gradually became more generalized.

In a Boston study, women with cancer of the breast elected to be treated by radiation and chemotherapy following minor surgery, rather than by radical surgery with eventual loss of the breast. Most of the women who refused radical surgery were physician's wives. Therefore, physicians must learn that women are as afraid of having a breast removed as they are of cancer itself. Preserving the limb of a child or a young person without compromising survival is a tremendous achievement. Hence, the optimal choice of management is to tailor it precisely to the extent and behavior of the tumor.

In California, legislation effective January 1, 1981 has added Section 1704.5 to the Health and Safety Code. This new law requires that breast cancer patients be informed by their physicians of the alternative effective methods for the treatment of breast cancer, explaining their results, advantages, and disadvantages. The physician's failure to so inform a patient would be grounds for charges of unprofessional conduct.

The multidisciplinary approach is a well-established new concept in which different methods of management are used in different combinations, according to the individual case. Surgery, radiotherapy, and chemotherapy are known for their effectiveness in the treatment of cancer; immunotherapy is still evolving. As for surgery, it may be more effective in some cancers but contraindicated in others, as in the treatment of lymphoma. Or, it may be equally as effective as another modality in, for example, the treatment of cancer of the head and neck. Other modalities are not without their limitations and indications.

All factors are to be weighed carefully to give the patient the best possible chance for more than just a cure. The most effective treatment regimen, either alone or complemented by others, is the essence of the multidisciplinary approach. One or more treatment methods will be planned according to the tumor's behavior and its actual or potential spread. Age, time, money, and the patient's desire to make a choice are all taken into consideration when two methods are equally effective. Knowledge of the presence of micrometastases outside the local tumor area, which are difficult to reveal, by conventional methods, has revolutionized the management of cancer. With the introduction of prophylactic management as a method of treatment, results have improved remarkably and survival rates have increased. In combining more than one treatment form in a course of management, the least toxic of each should be used to achieve the best results with the fewest complications. The dose of radiation must be changed; and the same concept should apply to surgery as well as to chemotherapy, particularly in the management of children. If long-term survival is expected, the chance another cancer will appear later in life or genetic mutation may develop, must be considered in this age group. Overkill of tumor cells by excessive management, disregarding the synergistic effect of all treatment methods, would increase complications and unnecessary mutilation without improving the survival rate further. A planned approach is designed from the start, and patient and family should be informed about the different phases of management. Any change from one treatment method to another should be carried out smoothly, without interruptions, with due explanation, and with previous knowledge of the patient and his family. If the patient is unaware of the following step in management, he might consider the new change an indication that his previous treatment was a failure.

Assistance Provided during the Course of Management

As problems are to be expected to occur during management, depending on its duration and the burden of treatment, outside help may be required and should be provided to patients and their families. At Stanford University, a short 6-hour course was given to tide families, with different problems, over critical times. The course was found to be very helpful to assure uninterrupted medical care to all patients. Discussions of the progress of management from time to time create good rapport with patients and their families. Feeling neglected by one's physician or deserted by family should be promptly remedied and is best avoided. A physician, just by being a good listener to the patient and his family, can be of great help to them.

How Much Should the Patient Know about His/Her Disease?

A patient's need to know about his/her disease is variable and controversial; the impact this information may have varies remarkably from one patient to another. Families react differently; their reactions are shaped by culture, social class, financial status, and other factors. Some families try to be protective and isolate the patient from reality. It is much too unrealistic for a patient to go through a prolonged course of treatment, which may last for many weeks, without knowing the nature of his disease. It is a great burden to place on the physician who is expected to deal with a family that has 'built a fence' around a patient; a well-informed patient is much easier to manage.

The patient and his family can be helped to develop a more positive attitude. A study in the Oncology Clinic at Temple University Hospital in Pennsylvania attempted to assess the family's readiness to receive information and their possible reactions. An estimated 81% of the patients stated that they had heard very little or nothing about the nature of cancer, and their acceptance of facts was difficult to assess. Some knew that they had had relatives who died of cancer and that it is a debilitating disease; others were afraid to learn about it and still others only wanted to know the positive things about cancer. Only 11% were dissatisfied with the knowledge they had about the disease and wanted to know more because, as they said, they cannot fight something they know so little about. Some patients even wanted to play a positive role in fighting cancer as their participation motivated them and elevated their morale. They felt they should be treated as persons, not as statistics of a disease. More knowledge was found to help both the patient and his family.

Changing Concepts about Cure and Failure

Better cancer management has reached a limit that requires more than just providing definitive management. To heal the person as a whole and not just his physical ailment is the goal. The patient's body, mind, and psychologic makeup are essential components of proper management. Success in treating a cancer patient is relative. It is not considered complete success to cure a cancer patient if, at the same time, that patient loses the ability to function further or to proceed with a normal life. By the same token, the concept of failure is also changing as it is considered a relative success if a patient lives with his disease, without remarkable symptoms, for 4 or 5 years or even longer. This is why palliation is considered an essential part of cancer management and should be a major consideration in decisions. This may be very much appreciated by patients and their families, as the quality of life is definitely improved, and survival prolonged without further pain, shortness of breath, or bleeding. Palliation is worth offering a person who is living a miserable life because of his disease. The length of palliation however, may be surprisingly extended and may reach years.

Palliative management varies from one person to another, but sometimes plans reach radical limits. Skill and experience are very much required and are helpful in planning a course of palliation. A pessimistic attitude is most often a result of inexperience and the nonrealization of the wonderful and dramatic effects of palliation. Therefore, a multidisciplinary approach should be considered in the management of palliation. Success in the treatment of a cancer patient is sometimes felt rather than measured.

The Five Goals of Radical Management

(1) The highest chance of cure.
(2) Preserve function.
(3) Best cosmetic results.
(4) Lowest morbidity.
(5) Rehabilitate the patient to resume normal life.

There are few examples to demonstrate the changing management of cancer in different locations. At present, treatment of cancer of the breast is undergoing a tremendous change with less radical surgical procedures – in which the breast is not removed – in combination with other modalities. Management of cancer of the prostate is also done by a course of radical radiotherapy so that the bladder's sphincter function is preserved and the loss of potency is less than with surgery [7, 9]. Breakthroughs in the treatment of leukemia and lymphoma followed a better understanding of the behavior and distribution of these diseases and prophylactic aggressive management by new combinations of chemotherapy and radiotherapy.

Varied Roles of Different Management Modalities

Surgery

Surgery is the major diagnostic procedure in almost all cancers. Tissue specimens should be available for microscopic study except on rare occasions, as management depends on pattern, differentiation, and other histologic findings. Radical cure of localized lesions with no existing or potential spread to regional or distant areas is ideally treated by surgical excision, as it is the most expedient modality if no mutilation is involved. Prophylactic surgery has its indications with oophorectomy and adrenalectomy. Surgery to debulk tumors or release pressure is also a good palliative procedure; decompression laminectomy or a bypass procedure with an obstructive lesion give dramatic palliation. A radical surgical procedure may be contraindicated in certain diseases known to spread widely and have multicentric locations, as in lymphomas and leukemias. However, surgery is now playing a role in the follow-up of cancer patients through what is described as second-look operations for the early detection of deep-seated recurrences, as is ovarian cancer.

Radiation Therapy

The value of ionizing radiation as an anticancer agent was realized soon after X-rays were discovered. They were first used palliatively for the treatment of advanced cervical and rectal cancers and produced favorable responses. At the present time, radiation therapy is very sophisticated with radiation-biology and physics constituting the basis for properly administering radical curative or palliative radiotherapy. Different megavoltage machines provide radiation to deep-seated tumors while kilovoltage machines are used to treat more superficial lesions. Brachytherapy, with the interstitial or intracavitary implantation of different radioactive sources such as radium and cesium which may be left permanently in the tissues or removed after a calculated period of time, is also available. In teletherapy the dose and size of the field as well as the number of fractions will depend on the intent of treatment – palliation versus radical cure – the stage of disease, and other pathologic details. It is usually aimed at the area of tumor and the region of potential spread. An advantage which cannot be achieved by surgery or chemotherapy is treatment of a wide local field. The therapeutic ratio is to be watched in order to give the highest dose to tumor tissue and the least to surrounding normal tissue in order to maximize antitumor activity while minimizing the dose to normal surrounding tissues to avoid complications. The tolerance of surrounding normal tissue should be carefully respected, otherwise resultant morbidity may be as serious as the cancer itself. A course of radiotherapy is given in a period of time that allows normal cells to recover and at the same time inflicts more damage on the cancer cells. Computers play an important role in planning and directing the beam and distribution of radiation within the body. High-energy photons, electrons, and heavy particles are used as each has its specific physical properties which are more applicable in certain situations. The patient must be immobilized and critical organs shielded so that treatment can be given every day for a prolonged course of radiotherapy.

Precise dosimetry, varying the shape of the distribution of radiation according to the geometry of the tumor and the location of critical organs, is administered using crossfiring beams. A prescheduled dose with the exact time relationship is usually worked out for the individual case. A slight modification is permitted according to the patient's response and condition. The patient should be assured that the procedure is not experimental; previous studies resulted in good survival rates, and as proved by animal testing.

The course of radiotherapy may take a few weeks and may be a heavy burden on patients and families, hence individualized care helps to tide them over this critical period. The obvious favorable response during management usually elevates the morale of sick people and their families. The reason for a delayed response to therapy should be explained to the patient with due assurance that utmost care is being given. It is essential that signs and symptoms complicating therapy be explained to the patient and family ahead of time as the patient may consider them complications of the disease itself. Medications to alleviate these symptoms should be provided.

Radiotherapy technicians play a major role in helping the patients during management because they are usually in closer contact with them. The patient should feel secure in their hands. Usually a good rapport develops between patients and technicians, which is usually long-standing. The technician's professional attitude usually helps avoid emotional attachments to patients, while the close working relationship between physicians and technicians helps them deal with problems as they occur during management.

Understanding the cell cycle of each tumor helps in timing the dose of treatment in radiotherapy or chemotherapy. Unfortunately, the exact duration of each phase of the cell cycle for each tumor is not known at the present time. The G_0 resting phase of the cell cycle can be very long, and usually the cell is at the lowest point of its sensitivity to drugs or irradiation; cells usually escape damage by treatment modalities if they stay in this phase of the cell cycle. Promoting the cells to proceed to a different phase of the cell cycle and synchronizing the time of their division are still to be achieved with different sensitizers. These drugs are presently used in limited quantities because of their neurotoxicity and other limitations [14].

Chemotherapy

The systemic effect of chemotherapy is exerted on cancer cells more than on normal cells. Unfortunately, the ideal drug – one preferentially absorbed by cancer cells, saving the normal cells – has not yet been discovered. Chemotherapy can use a single drug, but is given most often as a combination of drugs to potentiate their antitumor effects. Excretion of these drugs has to be monitored, and possible toxicity due to cumulative effects looked for carefully. In vitro assessment of chemotherapy before any given patient starts treatment, to determine its possible effectiveness, was presented by *Sidney Salmon* [10] at the 1981 American Society of Therapeutic Radiologists meeting. The tumor is first biopsied and cultured and various chemotherapeutic agents are assessed for clone formation. The predicted value of this in vitro response to chemotherapeutic agents was promising only in certain tumors. However, the in vitro growth capacity of many tumors is being improved.

Immunotherapy

It is theoretically possible to kill tumor cells and to do so with a high degree of specificity, without affecting normal tissues. It acts through a number of antitumor humoral responses and cell-mediated components, including a blastogenic response, a migration inhibitory factor, and lymphocyte cytotoxicity. Humoral immunity is theoretically the most effective modality with its three basic types: cytotoxic or nonblocking antibody effect, enhancing or blocking antibody effect, and cytostatic antibody effect. But the weak immunogenicity of antigens on the tumor cell surface (or sometimes the frequently antagonistic effects of the cellular and humoral arms of the immune response), the cancer patient's frequently impaired immunocompetence and the tumor cell's ability to break through the immune defense are partially responsible for failures. The antigen deletion rate of tumor cell replication, immunologic isolation, preemption and block factors also have a bearing on the outcome.

Why tumors are not rejected by the body's normal immune response was studied jointly by Beth Israel Hospital and by Boston, Stanford, and Brown Universities. It was speculated that tumors shed a membrane substance that promotes the formation of a fibrin gel 'cocoon' around the tumor, which acts as a physical barrier, isolating tumor cells from the rest of the body's immunologic defense mechanism. The tumor produces substances that cause surrounding blood vessels to leak a plasma protein and fibrin to surround the tumor, suggesting that an anticoagulant, to remove the fibrin gel from around the tumor might be therapeutic as reported by *Serena Stockwell* [12]. Cancer patients have a diminished ability to mount a delayed hypersensitive reaction or diminished T-lymphocyte response to mutagens in vitro. The different roles of immunologic reactions in host resistance to tumor growth were studied by *Biano* [1] and *Thompson* [13]. Immunotherapy could be achieved by passive, adaptive, active or semiactive immunization and nonspecific immune stimulation. The amount of free antigen known as the tumor load is critical and affects the outcome. *Biano* [1] mentioned that basal and squamous cell carcinoma of the skin are the first malignant tumors to have actually been cured by immunotherapy. *D. Chassoux et al.* [2] reported that experience with immunotherapy is very limited and that tumors with a mean diameter of less than 10 mm at the beginning of treatment are fully susceptible to the antituberculosis vaccine (BCG).

Lymphocyte cytotoxicity persists in the growing tumor, yet, at the same time, tumor-specific and nonspecific serous antibody blocking factors increase, as reported by *Stephens* [11]. Tumor-specific antigens (CEA) or blocking factors may potentially be used to detect human cancers such as colorectal cancer. Tumor-blocking antibody levels diminish after the tumor is removed so that a reduction in tumor mass has immunologic value, enhancing the effectiveness of subsequent immunotherapy by either stimulating T-cell immunity or reducing B-cell blocking activity. In addition, interferon has the capacity to inhibit the growth of a variety of tumors and works better with a low tumor burden, as reported by *Gressor et al.* [5].

Spontaneous Regression of Tumors

It remains to be determined whether the spontaneous regression of tumors is mediated by host immunologic factors, by intrinsic tumor cell characteristics, or by long-term tumor-cell dormancy. Neuroblastoma, a malignant tumor of early childhood, has the highest rate of spontaneous regression of any human cancer, according to *Gerson et al.* [4]. Spontaneous regression of this tumor correlated with lymphoid cell infiltration of the primary tumor and to the antibodies formed in the body [4]. Stimulation of the immune process as a possible explanation for most of the tumor regression was suggested by *Cole* [3] who reviewed a total of 176 cases of spontaneous regression reported in the literature from 1900 to 1964. The spontaneous regression of malignant melanoma is a well-documented phenomenon that occurs at the early stage of the pathogenesis of human melanoma. Spontaneous regression of metastatic melanoma occurs in only 0.22% of patients. About 40% of those with spontaneous regression have permanent cure with no relapse. Immunologic endocrine and metabolic factors may have a bearing on the outcome. In in vitro studies, blocking serum factors thwarted cell-mediated immune responses, but in animals whose tumors regressed, 'unblocking' antibodies were often found, according to *Hellstrom* [63]. Recent data have demonstrated that during the course of spontaneous regression, both nonspecific and specific cellular and humoral immunity directed at tumor cell membrane specificity are stimulated. In neuroblastoma, there is a positive correlation between the intensity of lymphocytic infiltration and the duration of survival, but no relationship between lymphocytic infiltration and metastasis. Sera of children with neuroblastoma contain complement-dependent circulating antibodies, cytotoxic against neuroblastoma target cells. Yet, the presence of such antibodies was found to be equal among patients with regressed tumors as well as in other patients.

It is suggested that perhaps an immune response may be responsible for the prevention of metastasis, even though spontaneous regression is possible in the presence of metastasis. After the primary tumor is resected in renal cell carcinoma and choriocarcinoma, occasionally metastasis was found to regress spontaneously. Interferon can retard the tumor's growth by acting directly on its cells, reducing their levels of DNA, RNA, and protein synthesis.

Hyperthermia has been associated with tumor regression and was studied by *Nathanson* [8], who reviewed the world literature. Spontaneous regression was found to be a well-documented phenomenon that occurs at every stage in the pathogenesis of human melanoma and appears to be a part of the natural history of this disease. Of the primary melanomas, 14.9% exhibited changes of blanching, pigmentation, and lysis of malignant cells in part of the lesion. In addition, unknown primary carcinomas were reported in 5.5% of 4,094 patients with metastatic disease, which may represent spontaneous regression of the primary tumor, even in the presence of viable metastatic cells. At least 33 cases of total regression of primary melanomas have been documented and reported in the literature. Spontaneous regression of metastatic melanoma was noted only in 0.22% of 4,541 patients. These patients had no obvious clinical features in common. Yet, the most common site of regressing metastatic melanomas is intradermal.

Hyperthermia, as a new method for treating cancer, is still evolving and is more applicable to the treatment of more superficial tumors.

References

1   Biano, G.: Clinical aspects of cancer immunotherapy. Immunity on cancer in man. An introduction. Immunology series, vol. 3, pp. 47–79 (Dekker, New York 1975).

2   Chassoux, D., et al.: Therapeutic effect of intramural injection of BCG and other substances in rats and mice. Int. J. Cancer *16:* 515–525 (1975).

3   Cole, W.H.: Relationship of causative factors in spontaneous regression of cancer to immunological factors possibility effect in cancer. J. surg. Oncol. *8:* 391–411 (1976).

4   Gerson, J.M., et al.: Neuroblastoma and host defense mechanism; in Oncologic medicine, clinical topics and practical management, Sutnick, Engstrom, University Park Press, Baltimore, pp. 61–70 (1976).

5   Gressor, I., et al.: Anti-tumor effects of interferon. Biochim. biophys. Acta *516:* 2131–2147 (1978).

6   Hellstrom, K.E.: Spontaneous tumor regression, possible relationship to in-vitro parameters of tumor immunity. Natn. Cancer Inst. Monogr. *44:* 131–134 (1976).

7   Hilaris, B., et al.: I 125 implantation of the prostate. Dose response considertations. XII. Int. Cancer Congr. UICC, Buenos Aires 1978, pp. 82–90.

8   Nathanson, L.: Spontaneous regression of malignant melanoma. 3rd Int. Symp. on Detection and Prevention of Cancer. Meet. Abstr. p. 317 (1976).

9   Perez, C.A., et al.: Radiation therapy in the definite treatment of localized carcinoma of the prostate. Cancer, N.Y. *40:* 1425–1433 (1977).

10 Salmon, S.: Predictive value of in vitro response of primary explants of human tumors to chemotherapeutic agents. Abstr. ASTR (1981).

11 Stephens, F.D.: Tumor immunology – a review of the present situation with particular reference to solid tumor and surgical implication. Aust. N.Z. J. Surg. *44:* 321–329 (1974).

12 Stockwell, S.: 'Cocoon' may protect tumours from immunological attack. Oncology Times *3:* No. 7 (July 1981).

13 Thompson, R.B.: An insight into cancer immunology and immunotherapy. Prog. clin. Pathol. *6:* 159–176 (1975).

14 Schuerer, E. van der: High dose multiple daily fractionation radiotherapy in combination with mizonidazole as a treatment of high grade malignant gliomas. A pilot study of the radiotherapy group of the E.O.R.T.C. Abstr. ASTR (1981).

Chapter 9

Medical Costs of Cancer Management

There is an increasing commitment to improved medical care by government, medical professions, and other agencies. The new objectives are to increase cure rates, achieve optimal functions and good cosmetic results, and restore the patients to their prior place in society. Consequently, medical costs are rising, especially in the management of cancer, which is becoming increasingly more sophisticated.

Cancer management is listed among the most expensive medical programs. Costs are similar to those for the treatment of alcoholism, benign inflammatory bowel diseases, congenital deficiencies, renal failure, and chronic degenerative vascular disease of the heart and peripheral vessels. The chief expense is repeated hospitalization, the cost of which is remarkably different from that for the treatment of other diseases, which may require only one hospitalization. In 1978, an estimated $ 192 to 194 billion were spent nationally on health care – 13% more than had been spent in 1977; per capita this amounts to $ 860.00. Spending for Medicare is doubling every 4 years because of increased medical costs and the graying of our society, reaching $ 34 billion in 1980. In the United States, Medical costs have risen to 9% of the gross national product, double that of 25 years ago. The National Cancer Institute (NCI) budget has reached almost $ 1 billion and has remained at this figure for 3 years. The items of expense are listed as follows:

(1) Cancer causes, prevention, and research.
(2) Detection and diagnostic research.
(3) Treatment research.
(4) Cancer biology.
(5) Cancer centers support.
(6) Research manpower.
(7) Construction.
(8) Cancer control.

Debates over these costs were studied by *Maloney and Rogers* [2] with the growing conviction that medical technologies are a major contributor, particularly with the remarkable advance in biomedical knowledge. A report by the Robert Wood Johnson Foundation indicated that even if the annual operating costs of the four widely used technologies – CAT scan, electronic fetal monitor, coronary bypass, and renal dialysis – were reduced by half, the net saving would be less than 1% of the national health care expenditure of 1978. The impact of these technologies on the total hospital cost was only 1.2% of the 13.4% increase in costs from 1964 to 1973. If the price of labor and other operating costs are added, the total cost of new capital equipment and its annual operation rises to above 15% of the national annual increase. The price of all existing CAT-scan equipment at $ 750,000 per unit is only 0.5% of the nation's 1978 medical bill. The study suggested that the big technologies help promote health care, particularly for the early detection of cancer, and should not be curtailed. The misuse of these facilities is probably what needs to be regulated. However, the statewide program to limit hospital costs by regulating large technologies has not produced substantial savings.

The leading category of health expenditure is private spending and the number of services provided to the patient. This is caused by the collective cost of thousands of minor medical tests and procedures for different individuals, which account for most of the annual growth of medical expenditure. A study by *Scitowsky, McCall et al.* [5] found that the number of laboratory tests in treating uncomplicated appendicitis rose from about 5 in 1951 to 30 in 1971. Tests per maternity case grew from 5 to 14 over the same period [5]. Attempts to control health costs have been discouraging. At present, recommendations to improve state programs include imposing limits on the use of small technology. The nation's yearly bill for operation clinical laboratory tests far exceeds that of the cost for capital equipment purchased by hospitals.

One study of the hospital cost of purchasing capital equipment estimated that approximately $ 600 million was spent nationally for large items. By comparison the bill for laboratory studies increased by an estimated $ 1 billion that same year. *Cost-effectiveness* is the issue. In the past, hospitals were encouraged to purchase and rapidly make available new technology to update medical management. The time may have come when ways may have to be found to make physicians more discerning in their daily use of such technology. The question is: Does the increase in small technology parallel the benefits accrued? The practice of defensive medicine shares a good part of the blame. Physician's reimbursements may be directed in a way to encourage them to be selective in their use of technology. In the past, favorable reimbursement for technology served an important purpose in encouraging physicians to master specialized areas and to incorporate the latest innovations into their practices. The time has come to swing the pendulum in the opposite direction to coax physicians to use their time more economically. Physicians must maintain a high-technology practice in their specialty fields, and it is entirely up to the physician to determine when and where to apply high technology. The notion that only a small segment of the medical profession is responsible for the excessive use of technology is incorrect. The system encourages physicians to overuse technology. Moreover, the system entices physicians to enter specialty rather than general practice.

Physicians' fees did not seem to add to the inflationary cost of medicine, as they rose only by 4% in 1979, which was below the rise of the general economy that year. In 1978, they rose by 8.1% when all items in the consumer price index rose by 9%. For the 12-year period 1968–1979, physicians' service costs rose an average of 7.8% annually, with 7% for all items and 7.7% for all services. Technology reimbursement seemed to increase more rapidly year after year than the increase in physician's payments, and this disparity is found to be growing even more. Between 1975 and 1978, the procedures reimbursed by Blue Shield of Washington, D.C., increased more than 50% whereas reimbursement for physicians' time spent increased only 20%. We must remember that cost of medical technology appears to have quite an effect on a physicians' style and scope of pratice, or even on his decision to seek subspecialty training. The problem in the use of technology is that it enables physicians to triple their income by applying a higher style of technology. This is far more income than that derived by using one's head and hands for the same time spent. *Schroeder and Showstack* [3] have shown how a physician could increase an annual net income from $ 31,000 to $ 90,000 by adding a number of quite defensible procedures and tests to the standard workup.

Insurance reimbursements should be redesigned to encourage hospital staff and private practice physicians to reduce the collective cost of their standard use of technology. Estimates of the potential national savings for nationwide incentives to reduce technologies exceed $ 6.5 billion from office visits to private physicians alone.

Merely lowering the physicians' income would hardly change the size of the national medical bill because reducing the physician's income by 20%, only reduces the national expenditure by 4%. Furthermore, a physician's fear of a low income might actually lead him or her to substantially increase the use of technology, as happened in West Germany when physicians wanted to maintain their current income level despite a 25% reduction in the number of patients seen. The accompanying cost, when physicians apply more technology, far exceeds the income a physician derives from having the tests ordered, because they include the cost of personnel required to run the tests, facilities to house the equipment, and additional operating costs.

It would be wise if a fundamental shift was made in medical education to teach students the discriminating use of selective diagnostic and therapeutic procedures. This limited use must be ingrained early in the medical career. The overall purpose is not to go back to the practice of old-time medicine, but to spearhead teaching towards the less costly use of available medical technology. At the Medical College of Ohio University, an education program was launched to reduce the overuse of diagnostic tests. If attention is paid to these issues and they are added to the medical curriculum today, their effect may reach 40% of the cost in a doctor's practice after 15–20 years. Patient referral by a general practitioner, to an array of subspecialists, would add to the total cost, particularly if the referral was not well planned or was not supervised by only one physician. The integration of services between general practitioner and subspecialists would avoid the unnecessary repetition of tests and any delay in the early discovery and management of the disease. Reeducating professionals and paraprofessionals and orienting them to specific cancer problems would help to reduce their management costs. Educating people to seek medical help early for their problems would also reduce the total cost of management. The cost of overexpenditure seems to extend beyond that by hospitals and physicians. There is a definite relationship between the life-styles and habits of people and the cost of health care. Alcoholics, for example, usually present with late cancer of the oral cavity due to the numbing effect of alcohol. Heavy smokers usually present with cancer of the lung at a late stage, which is mostly symptomatic and caused by the confusion between symptoms of cancer and what is described as smoker's cough.

The voluntary efforts of hospitals to reduce the increase in expenditures have resulted in savings by group purchases and various arrangements between separate community hospitals. More efficient inventory and attrition in the work force would ensue. A growing number of hospitals are developing cooperative relationships on an informal basis, which involves sharing equipment or services. According to American Medical Hospitals, more than 80% of the nation's hospitals share at least one service. Sophisticated technology and specialized financial management have pushed the new trend toward cooperative ownership. The management of two or more hospitals has increased from 1,315 in 1975 to 1,800 in 1979, which is a 37% increase and represents one-third of the nation's 6,000 community hospitals. Consolidation of hospital services, if accomplished by following the Federal Health Planning Guidelines, will not do very much, according to *William Schwartz* of Tufts School of Medicine and *Joskow* of MIT [4]. Both studied hospital beds, CAT-scan, open heart surgery, and cardiac catheterization as well as radiotherapy. The resultant savings were $ 1 billion after the guidelines were followed, which is less than 2% of hospital expenditures. It may be that comprehensive cancer centers manned by board certified specialists, aided by a tumor registry, and tumor board under the guidance of a cancer committee, with multidisciplinary approaches to cancer management, are two steps in improvising and consolidating cancer management between different hospitals.

The problems of fewer comprehensive regional centers located in only a few places would increase the burden on families during the prolonged course of cancer treatment and would adversely affect their socioeconomic status thereby increasing the psychological burden on patients and their families.

Isolating cancer patients from their families during management would impose additional psychological problems on them. A home away from home during management is not an ideal solution and is not without financial implication. More centers within different areas should be distributed among different community hospitals, depending on the size and range of their activities. One of the advantages of treating patients in community hospitals is to eliminate the fear they usually face when they are treated in hospitals known as cancer centers. These centers impose additional emotional stress, particularly on those who would not like to reveal their diagnosis to others. Even a cancer floor in a general hospital has its pros and cons. One advantage, however, of cancer floors is the availability of specialized nurses familiar with different cancer problems. Another is the presence of different facilities with the specialized technicians cancer patients need. The large centers at universities and different institutes are devoted mainly to advancing technology and education, but are used more for research purposes and initiating protocols for cancer management which, preferably, should be conducted at the large centers.

Another aspect of the hidden costs of medical care is the money spent on different programs, particularly if these are not well planned or controlled. Planning grants to assist health needs and to devise local projects that later acquire a national pattern have their proponents. The prospective randomized clinical trial is a breakthrough in medical research, as it entails harmony between different centers to achieve results in a shorter period of time because greater numbers of patients are managed with the same modality of treatment. The basis for a well-designed clinical trial should be set, according to previously obtained, solid pertinent data. The participation of different large centers helps to include enough patients to give studies statistical validity. The problem with these clinical trials is that they do not escape the self-selection problem and an inordinate length of time is usually taken to update information. The criticism of expanding clinical trials to community hospitals entails what were described by *Friedell* [1] in *Oncology Times* as 'bird dog' problems. A totally dedicated individual is needed, whose only job is to assure compliance to all details of different protocols by physicians at small centers. The participation of these centers may not seem necessary, but facilitated communication and sharing research knowledge may be an alternative. Some regard the clinical trials as expensive and limited in their scope since they can furnish partial answers to many questions. Moreover, clinical trials are viewed as being in the way of local free stands on different issues, which may be more helpful to different communities who may prefer to devise their own local projects. Their contention is that inclusion of small centers in clinical trials would add extra cost to the already burdensome expense of cancer management. They further claim that physicians are not taught to proceed with clinical trials, particularly if the trials are poorly designed and loosely conducted. Moreover, the hypothesis for these studies comes from retrospective studies and animal research and still needs to be proved. Grants to improve health needs and to devise local projects may be required more than just developing one national pattern for a certain management. But whatever is designed or chosen, the effectiveness of different oncology procedures as assessed by different studies, whether the results agree or not, should be pooled for further evaluation.

Health Insurance

At the present time, the cost of cancer management is a heavy burden of families, adding a serious impact to the trauma already present. Health insurance does not cover expensive cancer management and, as reported and confirmed by the US Congress, very little coverage is offered. There is a growing feeling that the nation's health resources must focus on heart disease and cancer, which together account for 70% of the deaths in the United

States. Others feel that health insurance covering cancer management should not jeopardize the fiscal standing of already existing health programs. Currently, programs are evolving that propose to cover catastrophic diseases. Catastrophic cancer health insurance allows the patient to afford the cost of cancer treatment. It would encourage cancer patients to seek early advice with the disease at a curable stage without any reluctance or wasted time because of the fear of impending costs. Reimbursement systems and federal taxation should be promoted in the direction of relieving medical costs, particularly for cancer patients. Moreover, payments for cancer patients from insurance companies should be expedited. Health insurance spending on the whole can be remarkably diminished as was done in a California institution where employees were reimbursed for certain amounts of money if they did not use health insurance services the previous year. This will eventually decrease the money spent unnecessarily for minor ailments.

There are other suggested strategies to decrease the cost of health spending:

(1) Limiting basic medical research would be an unwise step because of the major contribution that may come from unfocused basic science. Medical progress does not proceed in a single straight line, but depends on the integration of various bits of knowledge obtained from a wide variety of small pieces of information. To apply any restriction might seriously limit medical progress of unforeseen benefit to future generations.

(2) Cost-benefit studies should give priority to the development and distribution of technologies, particularly those that yield the greatest surplus of benefits over cost. The technologies that might save the life of aged persons or a limited number of citizens may be of less benefit than those that are more useful to a larger percentage of the population, particularly more highly paid young workers. Clearly, such cost-effect principles would have obvious overtones unacceptable to most Americans, as costs are considerably easier to measure than benefits. Many of society's most cherished values are not well suited to that sort of analysis.

(3) Limiting the distribution of large technologies according to population and epidemiologic characteristics. Costly machines that do not service many people have to be located in fewer centers. The problems of developing standards for thousands of items with smaller prices seem to be very difficult and do not serve any effective purpose in cost reduction.

(4) Eliminiation of the use of technology which does not carry any clinical value.

(5) Reimbursement for technologies should be given only if they are used according to specific guidelines and protocols.

(6) Unification of efforts of different cancer programs, duplication of the same services is costly. Volunteer work also helps decrease the cost and is appreciated.

(7) A drive to improve general health should be encouraged and incentives should be provided for nonsmokers or those who lose weight and to those who abstain from alcohol abuse. It was found that medical services for alcohol abusers cost 1½ times more than services for others. They accounted for 13% of a patient's use of medical and hospital services.

References

1   Friedell, G.H.: Bird dog. Oncology Times *3:* No. 2 (January 1981).
2   Maloney, T.; Rogers, D.: Medical technology. A different view of the contentious debate over costs. New Engl. J. Med. *301:* 1413–1419 (1979).
3   Schroeder, S.A.; Showstack, J.A.: Financial incentives to perform medical procedures and laboratory tests: illustrative models of office practice. Med. Care *16:* 289–298 (1978).
4   Schwartz, W.B.; Joskow, P.L.: Sounding board. Medical efficacy versus economic efficiency. A conflict in values. New Engl. J. Med. *299:* 1462–1464 (1978).
5   Scitowsky, A.A.; McCall, N., et al.: Factors affecting the choice between two prepaid plans. Med. Care *16:* 660–681 (1978).

Chapter 10

Returning the Cancer Patient to Society

Rehabilitation

This is a new concept that carries cancer management beyond the scope of definitive treatment; it is based on the realization that cancer problems are not limited to the cure of physical illness. The needs of cancer patients go beyond the excellence of medical or surgical care. Restoring impaired function, substituting devices to provide optimal function, and the best cosmetic results should be attempted. The perfect goal – resumption of regular activities – requires physical, mental, emotional and vocational rehabilitation. As years are added to a patient's life, it is equally important to add life to those years, and rehabilitation helps to make life after cure worth living. A rehabilitated patient who resumes his former position in society is an ideal witness to the vincibility of cancer and, as the numbers of these patients increase, the psychologic atmosphere surrounding cancer will gradually disappear. Physicians must know their patients and their potential problems before lines of definitive management are set. In a sketchy way future plans are discussed with the patient and his or her family. Subsequent to that discussion different phases of management are explained and in due time the patient is referred from one specialty to another. After definitive treatment has been completed, the transition from hospital to home should occur smoothly with no interruption in medical care. A plan to *discharge the patient* should be worked out with the family, with the patient's needs considered. Early discharge has its benefits because of the emotional gain as the patient returns to a family atmosphere and home-cooked meals, which eventually help to enhance his recuperation [1]. It also has financial benefits: a decrease in the number of days in the hospital is reflected in the total medical cost.

A home care program should follow hospitalization without interruption. This also contributes to a decrease in medical costs, which average $ 256.000 per patient per day. However, the cost-effect value should be carefully weighed when considering home care. This care must be comprehensive, provided by a team of different specialists – nurse oncologist, visiting home nurse, social worker, physical therapist, speech therapist, enterostomal therapist, orthotist, prosthetist, occupational therapist, and usually a hospital-based moderator – working together harmoniously. Psychiatric and other medical services are also provided. The services are tailored to the patient's needs and usually vary with age, sex, psychosocial problems and prognosis. A vital objective of the home-care program is to help the patient achieve *self-care,* to which he or she should be motivated as early as possible before dependency is created or an existing emotional condition is aggravated by different problems. Education and continued guidance are also offered, and the patient is encouraged to participate. He or she may be reluctant or afraid to become involved, or may sometimes be confused as to how to handle the new situation alone. With assistance, returning feelings of independence gradually replace the patient's earlier feelings of helplessness. Rehabilitation should never be initiated after problems have already been created, as it may be interpreted by patient and family as some form of treatment for an unexpected failure.

Prospective interaction was reported by *Whitely* [12] to solve 63% of problems facing rehabilitated cancer patients and was more effective than later interference. Ultimately, rehabilitation is supposed to prevent complications or minimize their effects if they do develop. Before definitive management is provided, patients should be sent to rehabilitation centers to meet with specialists, discuss plans, and prepare a timetable for future services.

Under medical guidance, *Reach to Recovery Volunteers* can effectively assist the patient during the immediate postoperative period, boosting his or her morale at times of distress and acting as living examples of the curability of cancer. Patient self-determination is closely related to the degree of success, as the rehabilitation program does not end with the same result in all patients. For example: esophageal speech in patients with laryngectomy may sometimes become almost perfect, simulating normal laryngeal speech, perhaps of a deeper tone, but nevertheless hard to distinguish from a normal voice. Rehabilitation varies in its expertise and sophistication but usually parallels the degree to which cancer management is successful. More advanced and modern techniques are available to the affluent. In poorer societies, the methods applied are adapted to local conditions because of technical and financial problems and a lack of trained personnel. Also, not all local hospitals have effective rehabilitation programs. Funds are provided on federal and state levels, and profit as well as nonprofit organizations are prepared to help cover the large expenses of these programs.

The primary concern of all rehabilitation programs is to expand the types of professional medical assistance given the cancer patient at home. A nurse oncologist and a visiting nurse offer routine medical care, handling, at the same time, different emotional problems and calling for physician's assistance when the need arises. Family physicians are very helpful in providing medical services at home. In Massachusetts, mobile vans are equipped to provide – within a radius of 10 miles of the hospital – such services as counseling, medical examinations, chemotherapy, blood tests, intravenous fluids, blood transfusions, small surgical procedures, and portable diagnostic X-rays. *Follow-up clinics* in hospitals and offices help to assess the results of treatment and to select proper management procedures. They also help in the early detection of recurrence.

Continued psychologic support at home should be provided through psychologic counseling and other means. The patient's losses should be appreciated and his emotions legitimized. Physicians may act as psychotherapists handling different problems as they surface. In their study of group counseling. *Ferlic et al.* [2] compared 30 newly diagnosed adult patients with advanced cancer to an equal number of patients who did not undergo group counseling. These investigators noticed significant improvement in perception and self-concept in the group that was counseled. But again, the benefits of individualized care must not be overlooked. All patients do not readjust to normal living at the same rate. Personality, prognosis, degree of physical disfigurement, age, sex, profession all affect the rate of readjustment. It is usually a tremendous challenge, particularly to patients with an obvious change in body image and to those with a physical handicap or speech problem. *O'Malley* [7], however, found that psychologic judgment is not significantly related to the severity of physical impairment in survivors. A close family relationship as well as strong religious beliefs and personal philosophies help the readjustment process.

Vocational rehabilitation is a part of total rehabilitation and is provided by specialists, depending on the patient's needs, qualifications, and degree of physical rehabilitation. An act, initiated by President *Woodrow Wilson* in 1912, helped disabled people achieve suitable work based on individual needs and talents. With proper rehabilitation, a patient usually develops a positive attitude towards the future. Needless to say, there are changes an already treated cancer patient will have to make in his lifestyle. For example: smoking and drinking habits will have to be changed, and patients with tracheostomies must not swim or take showers. Also, as dry and dusty weather does not suit these patients, a change of climate may be necessary.

Certain rehabilitation problems need to be discussed separately, as they present specific interesting issues to the cancer patient.

The Amputee

Amputation is a devastating challenge and a traumatic experience that requires tremendous readjustment efforts, not only to the loss of part of the body, but also to a prosthetic device. A prosthesis is a mechanical device that supports the loss of an organ or limb and replaces its function. The design and manufacture of these devices have improved tremendously over the years. For example, at one time, an artificial limb would not be available to cancer patients for at least 18 months after surgery – a period during which different emotional upsets could develop. Today, the amputee can be fitted with a temporary artificial limb almost immediately after surgery, reducing the emotional and psychologic trauma associated with the loss of an extremity or extremities.

Prosthetic planning should begin at the time amputation is considered and should be discussed by the different specialists involved. Total cooperation between surgeons and the amputation team is imperative, and the prosthesis should be readjusted as necessary; and the patient must be closely watched for such changes as loss of weight or breakdown of the skin. Of all cancer patients who undergo amputation, 50–60% survive more than 1 or 2 years. Even with a temporary arrest of disease, any attempt to improve the cancer patient's personal independence and to start his effective return to the normal daily routine activities of life will enhance and improve the quality of that patient's life. The contributions of prosthetic research and bioengineering, in addition to having improved the training of prosthetists, have, as stated earlier, reduced the adverse psychologic effects of amputation and decreased the length of institutionalization; when function is restored early, the incidence of phychologic problems decreases. A temporary prosthesis can be applied as early as 48–72 – after surgery – with some variation according to age and general condition of the patient – making controlled weight-bearing possible. To tailor prostheses to individual needs, designers must understand surgical technique. Conversely, surgeons must be familiar with the different prostheses available and the degree of function each can provide. For example: myoplasty is a common procedure in which major muscle groups are sewn together over the severed end of the bone, permitting the muscles to contract isometrically, limiting their atrophy, and helping to pad the stump for better muscle control. As a result, weight-bearing is more comfortable, making early ambulation possible. This, in turn, is followed by less phantom pain, better patient motivation, and less psychologic impact. With early ambulation, the patient's general physical condition improves, motor coordination is maximized, wound healing is accelerated, and local circulation improved; less venous stasis and edema occur. A solid stump makes for a proper fit, which results in a better gait. Experienced orthotists and prosthetists should be available to the patient because gait education is a tremendous challenge. Consequently, reeducation by experts, with the help of available equipment, patient determination, and family closeness are needed to spur the patient's return to a normal life.

Laryngectomy

Radical surgery for cancer of the head and neck may have a devastating psychologic impact, threatening the socioeconomic security of the postsurgical patient who views his body as having been mutilated. Problems with verbal communication and the loss of special senses lead to various problems. Plastic surgery may be required before the patient can adapt to living once again. Behavioral changes vary markedly, but surprisingly may be minimal or absent. For laryngectomized patients, voice restoration can be accomplished either through an artificial larynx or esophageal speech, which may be excelled in some more than others. Laryngectomized patients are bound to be subject to severe distress and frustration because they are unable to communicate with others: they develop a fearful feeling of incarceration and exclusion from society. Other problems related to this stoma include dryness and crust formation. A close relationship with the family in addition to medical assistance, education and rehabilitation will not only help the patient but comfort him as well. Volunteers experienced with laryngectomies may also be of great help.

Colostomy and Ileostomy

A colostomy is a surgical opening in the abdominal wall, connected to the large bowel; an ileostomy is an opening connected to the small bowel. Convincing a patient to undergo such procedures is not an easy task as they usually are reluctant to accept a change that may compromise their daily living habits and jeopardize their lives. The problems of colostomy, ileostomy and ileal bladder are usually magnified by the opening in the abdominal wall. A full explanation of the implications of the procedure would convince the patient that it would be life-saving. Without it his life would be in danger, a situation far worse than the colostomy itself. It is usually looked upon by the patient as a nightmare and its impact is reflected in the patient's behavior, social contacts, and business relationships. Feelings of abhorrence and disgust are common and usually expected, as the patient watches his bowel or urine content come out of an opening in the wall of his abdomen. These feelings are more distressing if the patient realizes that the opening will remain with him for the rest of his life. The experience is not only upsetting to the patient but to his or her partner as well. Moreover, it is very embarrassing for the patient to associate with people if no previous instruction has been provided and no precaution has been taken to control the elimination of gas through this opening.

Great care is required to guide the patient through these difficult times to enable the resumption of normal life. Ostomy clubs for previously treated patients can, under medical guidance, provide a tremendous boost in morale, reassuring new cancer patients and giving them a new, positive outlook that enables them to resume their rightful positions in life.

Before aggreeing to undergo surgery, the decision would be easier for the patient to make if he or she could converse with a successfully treated cancer patient with the same problem. To dilute the trauma of the new experience, the patient should be prepared, in advance, for this new life. Even an adequate stoma in the unprepared patient may invite problems that could have been easily avoided by prior education and adequate explanation. Teamwork efforts should be started even before surgery; the complete cooperation and understanding of surgeon and enterostomal therapist, trained nurses, and members of ostomy societies are required.

Proper placement of the stoma makes function and management much easier. The opening in the skin should be away from the incision line and the umbilicus, iliac crest, rectus muscle, old scars, fat folds, or the radiation field. It should also be away from the waistline for ease in bending, particularly in young women who wear belts. It should also be placed away from other medical problems such as skin lesions or hernias, and its position on the skin should be marked by the enterostomal therapist so that the permanent collection apparatus can be fitted properly. The stoma must be visible and accessible to the patient. Later stricture, herniation, or an ill-fitting collection bag may delay the patient's ambulation. If the patient gains or loses weight, the appliance will have to be refitted.

Many of these difficulties could be avoided by letting the patient wear the appliance and become familiar with it before surgery so that he or she is assured the stoma will be placed in the ideal location and not interfere with one's clothing, movements, or physical activities. An enterostomal therapist can give helpful preoperative counseling.

In the immediate postoperative period, intensive nursing is required to assure the patient that the situation is manageable and to provide support at a time of extreme emotional demand. If no assistance or the wrong advice is given, the experience may be too traumatic for the patient to face alone. The postoperative period does not end with discharge from the hospital but extends to the early days at home. Continuous supervision and close contact should be maintained and the proper advice given continually. For example, if the lavage tube is introduced into the stoma improperly, it could perforate the bowel. In addition, proper timely irrigation every other day may restore voluntary bowel movements and give better control of bowel function. Ill-timed irrigation may lead to loose bowel movements so that the patient's clothes are soiled causing justifiable emotional upsets. The skin around the stoma should be cleansed and protected so that it does not break or become inflamed. If the stoma is proximally placed, the fecal contents are more irritating to the skin than if it had been located distally. Soiling of the skin would produce greater inflammatory reactions. Gas and odor are most embarrassing to patients socializing with others. Proper dietary habits, avoiding certain habits such as chewing gum or swallowing air would help to eliminate the gas problem. Foods that form less gas and which do not lead to constipation are usually preferable. Oral deodorizers also help. Patients should be warned against lifting heavy weights. It may be difficult for patients with meticulous habits to readjust, but most patients should be able to resume their normal social and business activities after a readjustment period.

Breast Cancer

Because of the complexity of problems inherent in cancer of the breast, not all women should be subjected to the same structured plan after mastectomy. No two women have the same outcome; various factors interact to shape the final picture. Sex life, family relations, future motherhood, clothing, and breast prostheses are unique to each patient and their management must be individualized. A certain amount of caution should be exercised before group therapy is prescribed. Age, self-motivation and mental attitudes must all be considered. One tremendous challenge facing a mastectomy patient is confrontation with teenage daughters, particularly those entering adolescence and beginning to develop breasts. Finding the right words to use to explain the breast loss is very difficult, and mothers need courage and wisdom to do so. In these cases, outside help is much appreciated. Great help should be given, immediately after surgery, to such a patient through a meeting with a mastectomy patient, who has gone through this experience and is finally out of the woods and who became well-adjusted to life. *Reach to Recovery* volunteers, who are part of the American Cancer Society, and members of different cancer clubs can offer, under medical supervision, this help. The opinions reflected in different studies vary as to the depth of post-mastectomy changes. *Lewis et al.* [4] emphasize the role of the appropriate individual to provide such support. *Woods and Earp* [13], in a 4-year post-mastectomy study of 45 women cured of breast cancer, found that these patients did not feel they had been properly prepared for the postoperative experience. In addition, they were not familiar with Reach to Recovery, a supportive organization. In his study of the psychologic implications of mastectomy, *Ray* [9] found that fear of loss of a breast and the possibility that the cancer will recur are reflected in significant depression, remarkably different in patients who have undergone other major surgical procedures. Conversely, *Worden and Weisman* [10] reported the fallacy in postmastectomy depression and denied the prominence of lowered self-esteem, increased health concern and loss of energy because of the symbolism and sexual significance of breasts. Comparing breast cancer patients to women with other cancers, they found that the difference in the incidence of depression was about the same; 20% of breast patients compared to 18% of others. They recommended self-hypnosis for women to promote enjoyment of physical contact with their partners, and to overcome physical pain, the feeling of rejection, or a poor self-image.

The problem of *breast reconstruction* is a relatively new and very critical one. Not every patient is eligible for it, particularly if there is a good chance of local recurrence or the patient has had an excessive radiation reaction or has tight skin. Breast reconstruction is only indicated if the possibility of tumor cell reimplantation is less than 5%. The reconstruction could mask a recurring tumor, according to *Randal and Guthrie* [8]. At no time should the procedure be done to satisfy sexual problems if it would compromise survival. Nipple reconstruction is done if the patient requests it. The full thickness of the labia majora or pieces of the opposite nipple can be used for the reconstruction. Of the 30.2% of 149 patients who had nipple area complexes, 50% were involved with cancer.

Other forms of radical treatment are available for women who refuse to have one or both breasts removed. Survival rates are comparable to those following mastectomy, with no additional complications. Radical radiotherapy for stage I and II breast cancers has resulted in comparable survival rates.

Problems after Penectomy

Patients with cancer of the penis are prone to emotional problems, and guidance and counseling are required components of total patient care. Psychotherapy – including marital and sex therapy – are an integral part of counseling. According to *Mathews et al.* [5], the treatment of penile cancer encompasses more than excising the lesion.

Maxillofacial Radical Surgery

With commando procedures and radical head and neck surgery, there is an accompanying change in body image and expected emotional changes that vary in severity according to the degree of deformity age, sex, social class and prognosis. In the analysis of *Murray et al.* [6] of the effects of early maxillofacial surgery on growth, function and body image over a 20-year period, in 40 patients with a wide variety of maxillary and craniofacial deformities, results were highly satisfactory as judged by patients, surgeons and psychiatrists. The concept of earlier operative intervention has emerged as an aid in unlocking growth potential, diminishing secondary deformities, and improving the development of body image.

The social adaptation patterns of 152 cancer patients – interviewed at the Roswell Park Memorial Institute in Buffalo – who were facially disfigured following surgery, showed that 86.2% had adapted to their disfigurement [11]. Superficial disfigurement was seldom a reason for not returning to work or for not participating in social activities with workmates, friends, relatives and society in general. Disfigurement also seemed to have little effect on their involvement in formal groups. The reaction of society to disfigurement was perceived as positive (although staring was commonly reported). The reason for this high level of adaptation was suggested as a need to maintain a stabile self-concept. Age was also a stabilizing factor. The older the person, the less emotional the impact; disfigurement seemed to be a more acceptable (positive) alternative to the threat of death. The patient was usually prepared for the confrontation with society during the short hospital stay. The thought that the disfigurement was acquired to save his life made it easier for the patient to accept.

Readjustment to Society and Work

After comprehensive management is completed, continued care is advised to help the patient face new challenges. The patient needs assistance in relocating himself to previous surroundings. Exhausted by previous management and discouraged by depression, the fears deep inside a patient usually surface at this time and are usually reflected in a negative attitude towards society. He or she may be unable to cope with problems and fail to adjust on their own. Wanting to be independent but embarrassed to seek help from others, they should be offered help and counseling to obviate any unexpected deterioration. A loss of previous skills or physical power causes the patient to feel insecure. Any disfigurement that cannot be concealed is an obstacle to the smooth readjustment to society.

Job Discrimination

This may be real or sometimes imagined. Of the cancer patients interviewed in a survey in Southern California, 13% were denied employment because of a history of cancer; and 35% perceived discrimination when they returned to work after successful cancer management. One worker mentioned that his co-workers thought he would be unable to perform his job without assistance; that he would be a burden to them and be absent from work more frequently. Yet, studies have shown that 44% of cured cancer patients had no record of absenteeism. Patients who need to go back to work and cannot rely on disability insurance are usually more anxious to do their work and perform as well as in the past. Unfortunately, some workers were assigned to lesser tasks, not based on medical background, or sometimes given less desirable work or less convenient working hours. The cancer patient's capacity is usually not compromised after successful management. On the contrary, they have been found to work harder most of the time to excel their co-workers, and they try to be faster to prove their worth. Fearing the financial crisis of being laid off, cancer patients performed beyond their working capacity both physically and mentally in an attempt to prove to themselves and others that their performance capacity has not changed. At times, patients reported that co-workers mimic them, especially those whose speech has been affected or if there has been a marked change in body image. Although 86.2% of patients adjust to their disfigurement, are eager to go back to work, and are able to participate in social activities, others were slower to accept such changes. On the whole, reactions from society towards disfigurement are perceived to be mostly positive, as with the deformities seen in veterans, which are appreciated and respected by everyone.

Future of Long-Surviving Cancer Patients

More survivors of childhood cancers such as Wilm's tumors, Ewing sarcomas and neuroblastomas are being seen today, giving rise to new problems. In a study of 36 men and women 21 years of age or older, who had been treated for cancer during childhood, *Gogan et al.* [3] found significant differences among patients who had married or who were engaged, compared to those who had not married. A comparison of physical limitations, visible impairments, and psychiatric adjustment rating revealed a remarkable improvement in the married group. The decision to father children was a medical one, and long-term survivors delivered normal children. As far as the incidence of genetic inheritance and the development of malignancies is considered, further studies are needed.

References

1   Endicott, J., et al.: Brief versus standard hospitalization, the differential case. Am. J. Psychiat. *135:* 707–712 (1978).
2   Ferlic, M., et al.: Group counselling in adult patients with advanced cancer. Cancer, N.Y. *43:* 760–766 (1979).
3   Gogan, J.L., et al.: Pediatric cancer survival and marriage, issues affecting adult adjustment. Am. J. Orthopsychiat. *49:* 423–430 (1979).

4   Lewis, F.M., et al.: Psychosomal adjustment to breast cancer, a review of selected litera-
     ture. Int. J. Psychiat. med. *9 (1):* (1978–1979).
5   Mathews, D., et al.: Counseling after resection of the penis. Am. Fam. Physician *19:*
     127–128 (1979).
6   Murray, J.E., et al.: Twenty years experience in maxillofacial surgery. An evaluation of
     early surgery on growth, function and body image. Am. Surg. *190:* 320–331 (1979).
7   O'Malley, J.E., et al.: Visible physical impairment and psychological adjustment among
     pediatric cancer survivors. Am. J. Psychiat. *137:* 94–96 (1980).
8   Randall, H.; Guthrie, J.: The case for breast reconstruction after mastectomy. Cancer,
     N.Y. *24:* 218–224 (1978).
9   Ray, C.: Psychological implications of mastectomy. Br. J. Soc. clin. Psychol. *16:* 373–
     377 (1977).
10   Worden, J.W.; Weisman, A.D.: The fallacy in post-mastectomy depression. Am. J. Med.
     Sci. *273:* 169–175 (1977).
11   West, D.W.: Social adaption patterns among cancer patients with facial disfigurements
     resulting from surgery. Archs. Phys. Med. Rehabil. *58:* 473–479 (1977).
12   Whitely, S.B., et al.: Identification and management of psychosocial and environmental
     problems of children with cancer. *33 (11):* 711–716 (1979).
13   Woods, N.F.; Earp, J.A.: Women with cured breast cancer, a study of mastectomy pa-
     tients in North Carolina. Nurs. Res. *27:* 279–285 (1978).

Chapter 11

Pain and Suffering: The Hospice Concept

The pain of cancer may be triggered by the primary tumor or its secondaries. Also, the complications of cancer management may have side effects that induce pain. When bone or nerve are involved in the cancerous process, pain occurs. Pleural involvement or invasion of the viscera may be a cause of pain. The pain threshold varies in different individuals; it may be high in some, who seem to control pain to a large extent without, or with the least amount of, medication. Others may fear drug dependency and delay taking their medication as long as they can bear the pain. Conversely, there are patients who fear pain and resort to the strongest medication at the slightest perception of it. In the long run, they may exhaust their means of fighting the pain and palliation may be difficult to achieve. The expectation of pain may increase the misery of some cancer patients. To wait until pain begins, before medicating the patient, may require the use of potent drugs, and some physicians believe less medication is required to prevent pain. In addition, preventing the pain saves the patient from experiencing it. These physicians administer medication at regular fixed intervals, around the clock, rather than p.r.n. or as needed. Tolerance to pain was found to vary with the emotions and the patient's physical and medical condition. It decreases as the patient's physical condition deteriorates and increases with improvement. The drugs used to control pain vary in strength and are prescribed according to the patient's need. They may be given by mouth or by the parenteral route, and dosage is usually titrated for the individual patient. The objective is to treat the patient with pain rather than to treat only the pain.

As previously mentioned, pain is easier to prevent than to eliminate. One of the worrisome things to patients is their fear of the return of pain, leading to anxiety and sometimes severe depression. Sedating with analgesics, narcotics, antidepressants, tranquilizers and sleeping medications all help to control the pain. Pain medication, if self-administered, helps make the patient feel independent, and therefore more peaceful and comfortable. Different drug combinations are known to potentiate each other. These provide the mercy cocktails used for severe pain in advanced cancer. In England, the Brompton mixture cocktail, which contains heroin, is known to relieve pain without clouding consciousness. It is currently being used successfully. Phenothiazine, chloroform and alcohol are known to be added to this mixture. The AHS cocktail contains liquid morphine, liquid cocaine, liquid codeine, compazine, sugar, water and gin. It is claimed to keep the patient awake but free of pain and depression. Sometimes euphoriants are added to these cocktails to elevate the patient's morale. Furthermore, there are no reports of patients who have taken these cocktails in an attempt to commit suicide. On the contrary, patients report that they gain weight and become more ambulatory. These cocktails are usually resorted to only when other simple medications are of no help.

The continued use of powerful narcotics may ultimately lead to a state of drug dependence, but some view addiction in cancer patients with severe pain as nothing to worry about as psychologic addiction is rare. Pain medication may have side effects that can be handled promptly. In children, pain is different, because they are unable to communicate and explain its nature and extent.

When pain is severe and impossible to control, more drastic measures can be used. These include nerve block, which is usually done by neurosurgeons or anesthesiologists. If a local nerve block has a temporary effect, long-term relief – a subarachnoid block, injecting alcohol, phenol, or supercooled saline slush – may provide significant pain relief for weeks or months. If pain involves more than one anatomic location, rhizotomy is resorted to with surgical interruption of the posterior spinal routes as they emerge from the spinal cord; this can be performed on both sides. To relieve intractable pain, a spinothalamic cordotomy on the contralateral side is the most common neurologic procedure. Intracranial surgery can also be done to relieve pain. A prefrontal lobotomy prevents the patient from recognizing the pain, but since it is a major surgical procedure, it should not be done to patients with a short life span. Radiation therapy is a good, effective modality for the relief of pain and is very often used to palliate cancer pain, particularly in bones.

Hypnotherapy in the management of terminal cancer patients, studied by *Grosz* [1], is known to be effective for the psychologic management of pain, but should not be considered an integral part of patient care. It is not always successful and should not be looked upon as a panacea or a last resort in management. Hypnosis has always been associated with mysticism, but science explains it as a natural human ability to alter the state of consciousness and with it a change in perception. People differ in their hypnotic susceptibility, but some claim that even patients with low susceptibility can benefit from hypnosis using methods that modify responsiveness to it. Also, the depth of hypnosis is claimed to have no effect on the analgesia induced. There are no unpleasant side effects and, fortunately, the patient does not develop tolerance to the procedure. Hypnosis can also free the patient from the anxiety associated with pain and from depression. Some recommend it be used as part of the patient's psychologic management. The patient can be taught to initiate and practice self-hypnosis, creating a mental image to help the relaxing attitudes. Family members can even be trained to participate in a patient's hypnosis so that he or she feels less helplessness and more security.

Musical therapy in palliative care, proved to be a potent tool for improving the quality of life. Studied by *Munro et al.* [5], the diversity of its potential, in the hands of a trained musical therapist, is particularly suited to the diversity of the challenges.

Meares [4] mentions meditation as a psychologic approach to cancer treatment.

Difference between Pain and Suffering

This difference should be appreciated in cancer patients, and the medical profession should be able to differentiate between the two. Suffering is most often associated with anxiety, depression, sleeplessness, and emotional distress. For example, a colostomy or tracheostomy, although not a painful procedure, may subject a patient to a lot of suffering. A change in sex habits or urinary incontinence, in which catheter voiding is resorted to, are in themselves dehumanizing and obvious causes of misery. To adapt or accommodate to these changes is a tremendously demanding task in which psychologic counseling may be helpful. Anger over increasing helplessness and dependence on others are causes of depression and sadness. Family closeness and a homey atmosphere with understanding and empathy, but no sympathy, can help to tide the patient over these times. Professional and paraprofessional help is much appreciated. The painful part of cancer is the continued gradual loss of gratifying human contacts, isolating the patient from the rest of the world, long before death. The dehumanizing process accompanies the prolonged management of cancer and begins with the gradual deprivation of family contact and a decline in friendly relationships, so that the patient gradually shrinks away from the world.

The Hospice Concept

The word hospice was used to describe shelters for travelers. Presently, it describes institutions that provide prolonged care for cancer patients. The idea of the hospice was first introduced in Britain at St. Luke's Hospital in April, 1975. It started with a pilot program, under the guidance of physicians, to provide care for the patients' physical, psychologic and sociospiritual needs. The hospital, as an acute care facility, is not adequately prepared to handle the problems associated with prolonged disease. In addition, hospitals are considered terrible places for terminally ill patients whose psychologic and social needs are mounting on top of a deteriorating medical condition. As a matter of fact, a hospital is the worst place for cancer patients to die because their needs at the time of death cannot be met there. The hospice provides a well-coordinated, integrated supportive effort that deals humanely with the patient's temporal, emotional, and socioeconomic problems and spiritual needs. Medical care is provided without interruption and continued as an emotional support to the patient until the end. Usually, a patient does not welcome the withdrawal of his private physician from his care since any sudden change has a negative effect and is an ominous sign to the patient. Denying further treatment should be done only for medical reasons. It should be waived with the utmost care, discussed with the family, and comply with the law. At no time should statements such as 'nothing further could be done' be made to the patient. Pain and suffering are no justification for such a decision, as they are obvious proof that the patient is still alive. What the patient actually needs is stronger pain medication. Discontinuing supportive measures should also be weighed with extreme caution. At no time should the patient feel abandoned or left to die on his own. Hope must not be withdrawn abruptly. The physician should never accept the role of an executioner making any decision not within medical and human grounds. Therapeutic murder is not allowed to end the patient's misery and the patient should never be considered a vegetable or nonperson except on a strong medical or legal basis. Euthanasia is against all human values, ethics, or religious beliefs. We do not give life, hence we have no right to take it away. The question of giving a patient experimental drugs should be discussed with the family after compliance with current regulations. False hopes should not be given to the patient or family as proper information and a realistic assessment of the situation enable the family to proceed with future planning.

One of the critical issues on which most physicians disagree is how much information should be given to a dying patient. Generally speaking, it varies with the personality of the patient and family guidance. Improperly provided information may have a negative effect on the patient and may result in a suicide attempt. Despite recent emphasis on the need for open communication about impending death between the dying patient and his family, different studies reflect various opinions. In a study by *Hartwich* [2] disclosing the diagnosis to a terminally ill patient was discussed and interviews of 56 subjects who had been 'told the truth' about their condition revealed that the effects of age, personality structure, duration of knowledge, social contact, and religiousness of the patient were reflected in the patient's ability to cope with the information provided. When the process of adjustment was assessed, *Hartwich* found that these factors provide optimum conditions for a positive adjustment when the diagnosis was disclosed. Advanced years, good social contact, and optimal non-neurotic personality structure have a bearing on the outcome. The presence of only one or two of these factors provides the conditions for 'telling the truth'. In a young patient with restricted social contact and who therefore has a more markedly neurotic personality, particular caution should be taken against disclosing the nature of the disease; otherwise, there is the danger of a negative reaction or a suicide attempt [2]. In hospices, more personalized treatment and supportive care are given. Family participation on a 24-hour-per-day, 7-day-per-week basis is allowed, naturally taking the patient's physical condition into consideration. Unlimited visiting hours to family, friends and even pets is permitted. At the same time, the patient's privacy is guaranteed, as no television cameras are allowed. A decision to admit the patient to the hospice should be carefully weighed by physician and family. A patient whose health is improving would be emotionally upset if admitted to the hospice unnecessarily. A patient whose condition was deteriorating should be moved out for psychologic and emotional reasons, if he begins to show signs of improvement.

Hospice work is particularly challenging to the nursing staff. Different assignments are very demanding. Handling wet bed sheets, bathing and cleaning patients, and helping them with voiding and bowel movements are laborious tasks. Feeding and walking them are added burdens to continued medical care. The emotional stress on the nursing staff is high and a lot of help is required to provide adequate care to meet all of the services. A nurse can be a giver and a receiver; ways should be explored to help them out. Strategies need to be developed and no doubt volunteers could be of major assistance. Otherwise burned-out nurses would be unable to offer patients the required help assigned to them.

A peaceful environment with a less institutional look is essential. The hospice offers flowers, a gift shop, a chapel, a garden, colorful clothing, clean robes, and a nice-smelling, well-ventilated quiet place. Different foods and pleasant eating places with good company and friendly talk help to decrease the institutional atmosphere. Even birthday parties shared with family and friends are encouraged. A living room for families, programs for children, and facilities for their long stay should be provided. Friends can be seen on a porch or solarium in order to have a few pleasant moments in a homey atmosphere. Good rapport with the patient and family is one of the main objectives at these times of emotional exhaustion. Another is that family problems also be taken care of. It is a great burden on any one person to handle the needs of a dying patient alone. Self-criticism may be reflected and may be severe on the family after the patient dies, and joint decisions would help to eliminate this after-effect and save them from self-criticism. A physician's contact with the patient extends to helping in the management of dying. The concept of psychologic adjustment to illness occurs to a varying degree in individuals and according to several conditions. According to *Marrow et al.* [3], a scale for assessing a patient's psychologic adjustment can be worked out.

The word 'terminal' is very depressing to patients as it signifies abandonment of all hope. The words 'advanced stage' may be preferable. One of the difficult tasks in the hospice is to teach the patient to accept death. Spiritual needs should be met and socioeconomic problems taken care of. It is very comforting to the dying patient to know that he or she is not leaving behind any problems; that everything is well taken care of. The patient's adjustments should be watched carefully until equanimity develops; acceptance will always come. It is a very terrible feeling to have a patient compare death to annihilation, as the existentialists believe that death is the most awful part of life. Death should be looked upon as part of living; it is as natural to die as it is to be born. With the help of religious beliefs, death is considered the beginning of a new and eternal life. The ancient Egyptians were very practical about life and death and prepared their dead for a new life after resurrection. In other traditions, death is celebrated as a festival, as life without death is considered to be incomplete. Some people prefer to die at home and it is important to plan for this; the patient has the right to die at home if he so chooses. Death with dignity and withholding further medical help are not synonymous with euthanasia, which is merciful killing or therapeutic murder. We should not dehumanize the experience of dying.

Hospice services may even extend to the period of bereavement as psychological and social problems continue to be distressing. The family's adjustment to life without the patient should begin before death and could be helped and guided by professional advice. Not all family members are expected to take stress equally, and the help offered should vary according to individual needs. Help given to families by involving them in different activities was suggested by *Vaohon et al.* [6]. Widows of cancer patients were compared with widows in general and to widows of men with chronic cardiovascular disease in particular. Of those who were told their husband was dying, 40% refused to accept the warning. Only 29% of the couples openly discussed the possibility of death. More than half of those who did not talk with the husband about impending death reported that this made no difference in their initial adjustment to bereavement. It was noted that for a woman the stress of her husband's final illness led to a specially different bereavement period. Significantly more widows of cancer patients than of patients with other illnesses perceived themselves to be in poor health during this initial bereavement period.

References

1   Grosz, H.J.: Hypnotherapy in the management of terminally ill cancer patients. J. Indiana St. med. Ass. *72:* 126–129 (1979).

2   Hartwich, P.: The question of disclosing the diagnosis to terminally ill patients. Arch. Psychiat. NervKrankh. *4:* 227 23–32 (1979).

3   Marrow, G.R., et al.: A new scale for assessing patient's psychological adjustment to medical illness. Psychol. Med. *8:* 605–610 (1978).

4   Meares, A., et al.: Psychological approach to cancer treatment. Practitioner *222:* 119–122 (1979).

5   Munro, S., et al.: Music therapy in palliative care. Can. med. Ass. J. *119:* 1029–1034 (1978).

6   Vaohon, M.L., et al.: The final illness in cancer: the widow's prospective. Can. med. Ass. J. *117:* 1151–1154 (1977).

Subject Index

AHS cocktail, pain control 134
Alcohol
    intake, upper digestive tract carcinoma 50
    pancreatic cancer 56
Alleys of cancer, asbestos 21
American Cancer Society
    antismoking campaign 77
    education, professional and lay 76
    Reach to Recovery volunteers 128
    rehabilitation programs 76
    research programs 76
    screening programs 77, 79
Amputation
    early ambulation 125
    myoplasty 124
    prosthetic planning 124
Anxiety and depression 47
Atomic energy, nuclear waste dumping 23

Barium enemas
    cancer of colon, diagnosis 95, 96
    recommendations for use 27
Behavioral changes, cancer patients 45–47
Bladder cancer, local problem 10
Breast cancer
    dieting 43
    mastectomy, reconstruction after 128
    Patient's Bill of Rights 103
    screening for
        mammography, hazards and recommen-
        dations 25, 82, 83
        self examination, recommendations 82
    surgery, role 68
    survival rate 3
Bromptom mixture cocktail,
    pain control 134

Burkitt's lymphoma
    clusters 29
    EB virus, role 29, 54
    malaria, role 29

Cachexia 36
Cancer phobia 1
Cancergrams, current research, abstracts 73
Carcinoembryonic antigen 96
Carcinogen
    chemical 18–22
    chronic bacterial infection 6
    inhibitors 68
    irritation, chronic 6
    nitrites 20, 55
    nitrosamines and nitrosamides 68
    occupational 21
    radiation
        mammography 83
        X-ray studies 23
Carcinogenesis
    cellular transformation 7
    genetic factors 29
    genetic mutation 8
    intracellular changes 7
    latent period 7
    promoters 50
    repeated insults by carcinogens 6
    suspected factors 4
Carcinogenicity, causes 19
Cervical cancer
    incidence 55
    Pap smears 89
    risk factors 87
    screening 79, 86
    teenagers 89
    venereal herpes virus as cause 29, 89

Chemicals
  carcinogenic and teratogenic 20–22
  etiology of cancer 5
  in toxic wastes, implications 19, 20
Chemoprevention, retinoids 67
Chemotherapy 109
Chest X-ray examinations 26, 40, 97
Clusters of cancer 1, 4, 22, 29
Colon, cancer
  barium enema in diagnosis 95
  fiberoptic colonoscopy 95
  high-fat, low-fiber diet in development 40, 91
  incidence 91
  precancerous conditions, detection 92
  screening 92
    hemoccult test 92
  sigmoidoscopy 94
  survival, increasing 3
  vitamin A deficient diet 40
Colostomy 125
Cosmic rays, radiation source 23
Cost of cancer care
  diagnostic tests, selective use 116
  hidden costs 117
  insurance 115, 116, 118, 119
  physician's fees 115
  services provided 114
  strategies to decrease 119
  technologies adding 114
Curability, factors involved 69
Cytology
  brush 95
  esophageal and gastric cancer detection 93
  sputum, lung cancer detection 98

Detection of cancer
  early, effect on survival rate 3
  screening programs, tumor size 9, 10
Diet
  cancer prevention 43
  gastric cancer 40
  high fat 39
  relationship to cancer 33
Dumping sites, teratogenic and carcinogenic chemicals 20

EB virus
  Burkitt's lymphoma 29
  spread through saliva 54
Education
  information centers 72
  lay public 69
  medical profession, role 72
Energy, tumor drain 36
Environmental chemicals
  cancer 17–21
  industry 18
  methyl mercury in fish, implications 19
  toxic waste 18

Familial cancer 20, 29–32
Family, necessary supportive role 34, 37, 45
Fat intake
  cancer incidence, effect 38, 39
  pancreatic cancer 56
Fiber, cancer incidence, effect 39
Fiberoptic colonoscopy, colon cancer, detection 95
Fiberoptic gastroscopy, gastric cancer, detection 96
Food additives, carcinogens 33
  see also Nitrites, Nitrosamines, Nitrosamides
Fungi, role in cancer induction 29

Gastric cancer
  cytodiagnosis 96
  fiberoptic gastroscopy 96
  immunodeficiency 15
  nitrite fertilizers 55
Genetic factors in cancer
  carcinogenesis, role 20, 29, 31
  gene mutation 30
Geographic variations 54
Guilt, factors causing 48, 49

Health and economy
  controlling environmental hazards 65
    risk-benefit ratio 65
Hepatitis, chronic viral, hepatocellular carcinoma 29
Hereditary cancers 10

High risk
  cancers as 20
  cervical cancer 88
  definition 78
  populations at 1
Hodgkin's disease, survival rate 3
Home care
  objectives 122
  post hospitalization 121
  psychologic support 123
Hospice concept 136–139
Hostility 48
Hyperalimentation 37, 38
Hyperthermia 111

Ileostomy 125
Immune defenses
  anticancer 12
  suppressed, cancer etiology 5
  tumor as antigen 13
Immunodeficiency
  cancer problem, role 14
  lymphoma incidence 15
Immunosuppression
  etiology of cancer 5
  medications, incidence of cancer 15
Immunotherapy 109
Incidence
  cancer of cervix 89
  cancer of colon 90
  cancer of lung, smoking 97
  changes, factors influencing 56
  geographic variations 54
  increasing, factors related 64
Induction of cancer, stages 22
Information
  American Cancer Society 76
  death certificates 72
  International Cancer Research Data
  Bank 73
  National Library of Medicine 73
  tumor registries 72
Interferon
  activity 111
  illegal sales, hazards 71

International Cancer Research Data Bank,
  see Information
Irresponsible journalism 71

Laryngectomy 125
Life styles, cancer 66
Lung cancer
  chest X-rays 26, 27, 97
  smoking 97
  sputum cytology 97
  survival improving 3
  vaccines against, studies 68
Lymphatic system, cancer cell invasion 9

Malignant cells
  behavior 8
  dissemination 11
  immunologic surveillance 14
Malnutrition 34
Mammography
  evaluation
    HIP study 82, 85
    potential carcinogenic effects 25, 83
    recommendations for screening 83
  guidelines for use 26, 27
  radiation exposure, hazards 26
  screening
    cost-benefit ratio 85
    detection rate 84
Management
  assistance during 104
  changing concepts 105
  chemotherapy 109
  costs 113
    strategies to reduce 119
      diagnostic tests, selective use 116
      hidden 117
  excessive 104
  Patient's Bill of Rights, physician's changing role 102
  radiation 107
  radical, goals 106
  surgery 106

Maxillofacial surgery, radical
  job discrimination 130
  social adaptation after 130
Mercy cocktails, pain control 134
Metastatic melanoma, spontaneous
  remission 111

Nasopharyngeal cancer
  geographic incidence, variations 54
  virus 29
National Cancer Institute
  education and training programs 77
  self-examination program,
    breast cancer 81
National Library of Medicine,
  cancer research, projects information 72
Neuroblastoma, heredity 10
News media, promoting fear of cancer 70
Nitrites
  carcinogenic, foods 20
  fertilizers, cause of gastric cancer 55
Nitrogen balance
  hyperalimentation 38
  importance 38
Nitrosamides, carcinogen 68
Nitrosamines
  carcinogen, foods 33, 54, 66
  gastric cancer incidence 55
Nutrition
  food in carcinogenesis 32
  good nutrition in tissue healing 34, 37
  malnutrition, hazards 35
  overnutrition, deaths related to 27

Occupational carcinogens, smoking 21, 27
Oncology overviews, abstracts of published
  literature 73
Ovarian carcinoma, surgery, precancerous
  lesions, role 68
Overweight, cancer 34, 38, 44

Pain
  control
    nerve blocks 134
    hypnotherapy 134
    mercy cocktails 134
    suffering, differences between 135

Palliation 105, 106
Pancreatic cancer 56
PAP smear, early cervical cancer detection 89, 90
Penectomy, problems after 129
Pollution biology 17
Prevention
  diet 40–43
  epithelial cell carcinomas 67
  goals 63
  vitamins 40–42, 67, 92
  see also Chemoprevention
Procarcinogen, promoters of cancer 50
Prophylaxis, see Prevention, Chemoprevention
Psychologic adaptation, ego strength 46
Public education
  medical profession 72
  need for accurate knowledge
    breast self-examination teaching 81, 82
    information centers 72
    organizations providing 76, 77
    publications providing 73

Quackery
  cancer patients as victims 74–76
  crusade against 74

Radiation
  ionizing, sources 23
  X-rays and cancer
    exposure during medical use
      mammography 25, 26
      safeguards against 125
      unnecessary 24, 25
      viruses 28
Rehabilitation
  goals 122, 123
  vocational 123
Retinoblastoma 10
Retinoids in cancer prevention 67
RNA tumor viruses 29

Screening for cancer
  breast self-examination 70, 81, 82
  cost-effectiveness 79–81

Screening for cancer (cont.)
  rationale 78
  requirements of programs 79
  sampling populations 79
  who should be screened 79
Scrotal cancer, occupational 21
Sexuality, cancer of sex organs 58, 59
Sigmoidoscopy, value 94
Skin cancer
  current facts 70
  survival 3
  ultraviolet and sunlight causing 28
Smoking
  campaign against 77
  cancer risk 27
  lung cancer, incidence 97
  occupational hazards 21, 27, 28
  respiratory tract, carcinoma 50
Stress and cancer 44
Suicide among cancer patients 49
Sunlight and skin cancer 28
Supplementary feeding, *see* Hyperalimentation
Surgery 106
Survival
  fighting back promotes 49
  increasing in cancer patients 3

Terminology, feat provoking 70–72
Thermography in screening 86
α-Tocopherol, cancer prevention 67, 68
Toxic wastes
  cancer 18
  chemical carcinogens and teratogens 20
  contamination of fish 19
  disposal 20
  nuclear waste dumping 23

Transfer therapy 37
Tumor
  as antigens 12, 13
  cells
    emboli 11
    fate in circulation 11
    shedding and dissemination 11
    surface antigens 14
    malignant, viral etiology 28
    multiple 10, 11
    registries 72
    spontaneous regression 110

Ultraviolet radiation, skin cancer 28
Uterine cancer
  local problem 10
  precancerous, surgery 68

Vaccines
  cancer prevention 68
  lung cancer, studies 68
Venereal herpes virus, cervical cancer 89
Viruses, cancer etiology 28, 29
Vitamin A
  cancer prevention 67
  colonic cancer, deficiency 40
Vitamin B, anticarcinogenic effects 41
Vitamin C
  cancer prevention 67, 92
  protection against gastric cancer 41, 42
  rectal polyps, effect 42
Vitamin E, cancer 41

Warning signs of cancer 70
Water pollution control 17–19
Wilm's tumor 10